AF825572

"BOSS Series"

Orthopaedics

Dear Reader!

We have produced another wonderful text "BOSS Series" on the Orthopaedics with the help of most experienced and versatile author R.N. Prasad. The author has taken great pain in making this book. The recent trend in PGMEE/ PGMAT examination can be successfully solved by reading this book. The chapters itself helps you to solve problem oriented clinical cases asked now-a-days in different PGMEE examinations of All India, AIIMS, PGI, State PGMAT, NIMHANS, BHU and many more like BPSC and UPSC etc.

Publisher

"BOSS Series"

Orthopaedics

R.N. Prasad
BSc (Dist), MBBS (Ran), MD (Pat) (Patho and Microbiology), DC Path (Pat), DCH (Pat)
Tutor-cum-Assistant Professor
Department of Pathology
A. N. Magadh Medical College
Gaya, Bihar (India)

Formerly Medical Officer
at Patna Medical College and Hospital
Patna, Bihar (India)

Ex-Tutor JLN Medical College
Bhagalpur, Bihar (India)

PEEPEE
PUBLISHERS AND DISTRIBUTORS (P) LTD.

"BOSS Series"—Orthopaedics

Published by
Pawaninder P. Vij

Peepee Publishers and Distributors (P) Ltd.
Head Office: 160, Shakti Vihar, Pitam Pura,
Delhi-110 034 (India)

Corporate Office: 7/31, Ansari Road, Daryaganj,
Post Box-7243
New Delhi-110002 (India)
Ph: 55195868, 9811156083
e-mail: peepee160@yahoo.co.in
e-mail: peepee160@rediffmail.com
www.peepeepub.com

First Edition: **2005**

ISBN: 81-88867-58-6

Printed at
Lordson, C-5/19, Rana Pratap Bagh, Delhi-110 007

to
the sacred memory
of
my father!

Preface

The present treatise under "BOSS Series" naming "BOSS Series—Orthopaedics" has come up to bridge the gap between those who are marathon runner to 100 metres. In fact it has come up also as per recently adopted MCI curricula and syllabus.

This book contains a comprehensive outline of the scientific principles and phenomenology that underpin the field of basic and organ-system orthopaedics. In each chapter, the author has attempted to highlight what are considered as the key concepts and pertinent facts.

The book is divided into several sections covering the whole of the "Orthopaedics" as per recent examination trends. This treatise has been made in such a manner that students will derive the enormous quantities of factual knowledge not only in Orthopaedics but in relation to *Medical Sciences* on the whole.

Besides that students will find it a useful guide to go through their *"University"* as well as "*Internal assessment"* examination (Viva-voice) quite comfortably fetching highest marks.

Lastly but not the least should be used by PGMAT/PGMEE service aspirants in understanding orthopaedics as a whole. Even practising doctors will find this book as a good companion to deal effectively with their day- to-day more complex clinical problems.

R.N. Prasad

Contents

Chapter one

General Consideration in Orthopaedics

You Should Know

1. The 1st bone to ossify in foetal life is—**Clavicle.**
2. Longitudinal growth is accomplished by—**Epiphyseal plate.**
3. Ossification begins in the foetus during—**5th week.**
4. **Bone matrix** is composed of—**90% collagen.**
5. When a muscle contracts the **Z bands** move towards each other.
6. Normal serum value of **alkaline phosphatase** in a 3 years old child is **5 to 14 Bodansky units.**
7. **Adult bone trabeculum** can be differentiated microscopically from **foetal bone** or **tumour bone** trabeculae by the **lamellar structure.**
8. **Collagen** is characterized by unique content of **hydroxyproline.**
9. The **osteoblast** produces collagen to form **bone osteoid.**
10. **Distal femoral epiphyses** are not seen before **35 years.**
11. The **precartilagenous analog of bone** arises from **mesenchyme.**
12. **Cartilage shows** extensive vascular channels in **embryonic life.**
13. The **total citrate in bones** makes about **45%** of the body total.
14. The **nidation crystal of bone** is calcium phosphate [$(Ca_3(PO_4)_2$].
15. **Synovial tissue** is **1st seen** in a **developing joint** at about **12th week of IUL/gestation.**

16. Most of the **joints** are differentiated and recognizable in a human embryo at about—**6 weeks of IUL/gestation.**
17. The **perichondral ring** is found around the epiphyseal plate.
18. The **suture** uniting the two parietal bones to the occipital bone in the foetal skull is LAMBDOID SUTURE.
19. The major vessels of the carpal SCAPHOID enter the bone at the distal pole.
20. In **hemophilia**, most commonly affected joints are **knees** and **elbows** joints.
21. Patients with MORQUIO's syndrome shows an **excess of keratan sulfate** on urine analysis.
22. The **viscosity of synovial fluid** is dependent upon the concentration of **hyaluronic acid.**
23. HAVERSIAN system are most perfectly organized only in the **3rd decade of life.**
24. A patients may **compensate for a short lower extremity** to equalize leg length by:
    - Flexing the knee and the hip on the normal side.
    - Walking on the toes tips on the shortened side.
    - Drooping the pelvis on the involved shortened side.
25. **Bone pain** originates from and is carried by:
    - Periosteum.
    - Myelinated fibres.
    - Blood vessels.
    - Unmyelinated fibres.
26. The **METAPHYSIS lies within the joint cavity** includes:
    - Upper metaphysis of femur.
    - Upper metaphysis of humerus.
    - Lower metaphysis of femur.
    - All the metaphysis at elbow.

*Note: The **metaphysis** that is not at all within the joint cavity is **upper metaphysis at tibia.***

27. **ARTHROGRAMS are especially useful in** diagnosing:
    - Loose bodies in the knee joint.
    - Congenital dysplasia of hip.
    - Rotator cuff tear of the shoulder.
28. **TELOGRAMS is a method of measuring** longitudinal length of long bone by radiography.
29. **Properties of bone collagen** include:
    - Only protein that contains hydroxylysine.
    - Glycine is present in larger amount than any other amino acid.
    - Exhibits 640A° periodicity in the mature fibre.
30. **Maturation of growth** is dependent upon a balance between thyroid and hormones from anterior lobe of pituitary gland.
31. HORMONES that influences **growth positively** include:
    - Thyroxine.
    - Growth hormone.
    - Insulin.
    - 17-ketosteroids.
32. **Synovial fluid characteristically contains:**
    - Fibrinolysis.
    - A dialysate of plasma.
    - Less mineral ions than found in plasma concentration.
    - More HCO_3^- and Cl^- ions than in plasma.
33. **Recognized effects of oestrogen deficiency** include:
    - Decrease in skeletal ossification.
    - Decrease in bone growth.
    - The breaking strength of bone is decreased.
34. **Recognized hormones that stimulate growth in height.**
    - Adrenogenic 17-ketosteroids of testicles.
    - Adrenogenic 17-ketosteroids of adrenal.
    - Hormones from the anterior lobe of the pituitary.

35. **Regarding the HAVERSIAN SYSTEMS of bones:**
    - Are most perfectly matured at age 24.
    - Become fragmented with the advancement of age.
    - Are directly associated with the remodelling of bone in response of physiological stress.
36. **Esterase, alkaline phosphatase** and **mucopolysaccharides** are the substances actively formed by **osteoblasts.**
37. **Synovial membrane** may contain normally.
    - Two layers of lymphatics.
    - Paccinian corpuscles.
    - A fibrocollagenous layer.
38. **Normal solubility constant** of **calcium** × **phosphate** ($Ca^{++} \times PO_4^-$) is about **40.**
39. **ANTALGIC gait** is a gait that is used to **relieves pain.**
40. **Steppage gait** is seen in cases of **peroneal nerve palsy.**
41. **Pain from colon and uterus** is referred to **low back.**
42. **Radioisotopes most commonly utilized for diagnosis** of bony lesions include:
    - **Strontium 85, 87 M.**
    - **Fluoride 18.**
    - **Gallium 67.**
    - **Technetium 99 M.**
43. The normal value of **Plasma uric acid** in the **male** is about **2 to 6 mg/100 ml.**
44. The **Carpal tunnel** is formed by the flexor retinaculum anteriorly and by the distal row of the carpus posteriorly.
45. At **birth** the **foot** is **flat.**
46. **Bars of cartilage** on either side of the neural tube fuse during the 4th month of IUL (intrauterine life) to form vertebral arches.

Table of Charts

A.	**Ossification centres and its appearance (age)**	
47.	Capital epiphysis of femur	By age one (1 yr)
48.	Distal epiphysis of femur	Present at birth
49.	Triquetrum	By age three (3 yrs)
50.	Capitate	By age one (1 yr)
51.	Lunate	By age four (4 yrs)
52.	Scaphoid	By age five (5 yrs)
53.	Capitulum of humerus	By age two (2 yrs)
54.	Distal epiphysis of radius	By age one (1 yr)
55.	Distal epiphysis of ulna	By age eight (8 yrs)
B.	**Bone/cartilage formation/destruction**	
56.	Chondroblast	Cartilage formation
57.	Chondroclast	Cartilage destruction
58.	Osteoblast	Bone formation
59.	Osteoclast	Bone destruction
C.	**Average age of closure of the epiphysis in males**	
60.	Clavicle	Over 21 years
61.	Proximal humerus	Age 18 to 20 years
62.	Marginal epiphysis of ilium	Over 21 years
63.	Ischium and pubis	Age 14 years
64.	Proximal femur	Age 15 to 17 years
65.	Distal femur	Age 18 to 20 years
66.	Proximal tibia	Age 18 to 20 years
67.	Distal tibia	Age 18 to 20 years
68.	Epiphysis of calcaneus	Age 14 years

Chapter two

Trauma or Hot Orthopaedics—General Consideration

You Should Know

1. **Single most important clinical feature of a fracture** is local bone tenderness/crepitus.
2. The **time required for healing of fracture** varies with—
   - Blood supply.
   - Site of the fracture.
   - Age of the patient.
   - Degree of soft tissue damage.

> ***Note:*** *It does not depend upon sex of the patient.*

3. It is true about **healing of a fracture** that:
   - There is initial hematoma at the fracture site.
   - Fibrous tissue replaces the haematoma.
   - Local acid pH facilitates absorption of bone from fractured end.

> ***Note:*** *It is not true that the* ***fibrous tissue*** *directly becomes bone.*

4. **Radiologically demonstrable calcification** and subsequent ossification occurring in the callus is evident in between 3 to 6 weeks following injury.
5. It is true about **healing fracture** that:
   - The calcium (Ca^{++}) salts are laid down in the osteoid tissue.
   - The tissue formed by the invading osteoblasts is termed osteoid.
   - The final stage of repair is the remodelling of the callus.

> ***Note:*** *It is not true that the haematoma is initially invaded by osteoblast.*

6. Radiologically united fracture is characterized by **bone bridging** the fracture not Haversian in structure.
7. Recognized F/O **consolidated fracture** include:
   - No pain at the fracture site irrespective of the patients activity.
   - Fracture gap is bridged by normal Haversian bone.
   - Radiological texture of the bone mass surrounding the fracture site is identified with that of the rest of the bone.
8. Regarding **fracture healing,** It is true that:
   - Rotation never is an acceptable deformity.
   - Shortening in minor degree at fracture site is acceptable.
   - Some angulation at fracture sites in children correct themselves.
   - The hyperaemia of healing causes stimulation of longitudinal growth.

> ***Note:*** *It is untrue that the fracture through epiphyseal plate causes bone lengthening*

9. The single most important factor in fracture healing is **IMMOBILIZATION.**
10. **Regarding healing of fractures,** it is true that:
    - No fracture unites in less than 3 weeks.
    - Fractures in adults take twice as long to unite as fractures in children.
    - Comminuted fractures are particularly slow to unite.

> ***Note:*** *It is untrue that transverse fractures take less time to unite than oblique or spiral fractures.*

11. **Delayed union** may result owing to:
    - Excessive movement.
    - Poor blood supply at the fracture site.
    - Interposition of soft tissue.
    - Infection.

12. **Non-union** is often seen in fracture neck of the femur.

> *Note: It is not seen in fracture mandibular condyle, Colles' fracture, and fractures of the 4th metatarsal.*

13. **PSEUDOARTHROSIS** is an recognised example of non-union.
14. Recognised fracture of **non-union** includes:
    - Radiologically visible fracture site.
    - Sclerotic bone ends.
    - Obliteration of medullary canal.

> *Note: It is not associated with absence of abnormal movement.*

15. Recognised F/O **Sudeck's atrophy** include:
    - Marked osteoporosis.
    - Vascular stasis.
    - Thickening of the soft tissues.
    - Pain.

> *Note: It is not related to undue joint mobility.*

16. **MALUNION of a fracture** is a fracture which unites in a position of deformity.
17. The bone area undergoing least corrective remodelling following fracture malunion in children is the **femoral neck.**
18. It is true about the **impacted** fracture of a cancellous bone that:
    - Presence of a zone of sclerosis at the fracture site.
    - Absence of crepitus and abnormal movement.

> *Note: It is not true that there is presence of callus surrounding the callus site.*

19. **In immobilizing a fracture,** both the joints above and below the fracture must also be immobilized.
20. **Regarding skin traction,** it is true that skin tolerates upto **8 lbs (pounds) of weight.**
21. The time period after which a **dislocated joint** may be expected to be **unreducible** by closed methods is approximately **2 to 3 weeks.**

22. **Prolonged immobilization of a** fracture patients causes:
    - Thromboembolism.
    - Skin necrosis.
    - Bronchopneumonia.
    - Demineralization.

> ***Note:*** *The least common problem associated with prolonged immobilization is stasis dermatitis.*

23. Through **skeletal traction** the **weight** may be applied upto **60 to 80 lbs (pounds).**
24. **Internal fixation** is useful:
    - In fracture neck of the femur.
    - In fracture of the patella.
    - In fractures associated with damage to vital soft tissues.
    - In elderly individuals.
25. **Prolonged immobilization** is associated with or causes:
    - Osteoporosis.
    - Soft tissue calcification.
    - Joint stiffness.
    - Formation of renal stones.

> ***Note:*** *It does not cause gallstone formation.*

26. The only fracture with a **bad reputation of non-union** in **childhood** is external condyle of the **humerus.**
27. **Indications for easing a plaster encircling a limb** may include:
    - Weak or absent pulse distal to the plaster.
    - Swelling distal to the plaster.
    - Increasing pain and discomfort at and distal to the fracture site.
    - Difficult or absent active movements of the muscles.
28. **Volkmann's ischaemic contracture** is a hazard of Plaster-of-Paris (P-O-P) splinting or cast.
29. **Fracture of a single metacarpal shaft** is satisfactorily splinted by adjacent soft tissues.

30. **Closed reduction** is impossible:
    - If the surgeon cannot obtain any purchase on one of the two fracture fragments.
    - If soft tissues interposes between the fracture fragments.
    - If there are several small fracture fragments around a joint whose accurate replacement is essential for the normal joint stability.
31. The **treatment of compound fractures** includes:
    - Wound toilet.
    - Use of antibiotics.
    - Reconstitution of skin cover.
    - External splintage with window or rarely internal fixation.
32. The **best bone graft for a case of non-union** is autogenous cancellous bone.
33. A **convenient site of bone for bone graft** is iliac crest.
34. **Fractures occurring in childhood differ from those in adult** in the following ways:
    - The fracture unite readily.
    - To some extent malunion can be corrected by growth.
    - The patient is usually unable to give any history.
    - The fractures may involve the epiphyseal plate and hence interfere with growth.

> ***Note:*** *It is not a fact that joint stiffness is common after immobilization.*

35. **Open reduction and internal fixation** in fractures ensuing in **childhood is never required.**
36. The **deformities due to malunion** in cases of supracondylar fractures of the humerus in childhood is best correctable by growth of a backward and angulation of the distal fragment.
37. **Shortening upto 1.5 cm** is easily tolerated in the lower limbs.
38. **Shortest stump for the forearm** is about **three inches.**
39. In **Syme’s amputation,** lower ends of tibia and fibula are divided transversely 3/4” proximal to the ankle joint.

40. Regarding the **technique of amputation:**
   - Nerves are best cut through with the muscles and left undisturbed.
   - The skin flap should not contain muscles.
   - Periosteum is divided at the level of bone section.
   - Muscles are divided half an inch below the proposed level of bone section.

> ***Note:*** *It is not true that muscles are sewn over the end of the stump.*

41. **Common sites of compression fractures** include:
   - The **heels.**
   - The **vertebral bodies.**

> ***Note:*** *It is not seen in the shaft of the* ***tibia*** *and the* ***metatarsals.***

42. The **management of a fracture** includes:
   - Reduction.
   - Immobilization.
   - Maintenance of muscle power.
   - Preservation of joint mobility.
   - Rehabilitation.
43. Recognised **causes of non-union** of a fracture include:
   - Anoxia.
   - Uraemia.
   - Infection of the fracture haematoma.
44. A **green stick fracture** is a fracture where part of the cortex is intact and part cracked. It occurs chiefly in **children.**
45. Important factors leading to **delayed or non-union** of fractures include:
   - Insufficient blood supply.
   - Interrupted immobilization.
   - Inadequate immobilization.
   - Shearing of rotational strain at the fracture site.
46. Recognised examples of **AVULSION fractures** include:
   - Upper pole of patella.
   - Base of 5th metatarsal.

- Lesser trochanter.
- Tibial tuberosity.

47. The **recognised criteria for implant materials** include:
    - Freedom from tissue reaction.
    - Freedom from corrosion.
    - Freedom from mechanical failure.
48. Recognised **causes of joint stiffness** due to fracture treatment include:
    - Osteoarthritis.
    - Intra-articular adhesion.
    - Sudeck's atrophy.
    - Myositis ossification.
    - Bony fragments within the joint.
49. **Recognised forms of traction.**
    - Skin traction.
    - Skeletal traction.
50. In a **compound fracture** there is a wound in communication with the fracture.
51. In a **subluxation, the articulating surfaces** of the joint are non-congruous and loss of contact is incomplete.
52. A **sprain** is an incomplete tear of a ligament or complex of ligaments.
53. **Stress fractures** are generally hairline fractures.
54. The average time for well-advanced **healing in cancellous bone** is about 6 weeks from the time of injury.
55. The commonest site of **myositis ossification** is the **elbow.**
56. **Delayed tendon rupture** is most frequent at the wrist after a **Colles' fracture.**
57. **Direct violence results** in **transverse fractures.**
58. **Indirect violence** will cause **oblique** and **spiral fractures.**
59. "Elephant's foot" appearance is due to **hypertrophic non-union.**
60. **Atrophic non-union** will cause narrow and rounded bone ends.
61. **Dislocation of the hip** produces **sciatic nerve palsy.**

62. **Fracture of the shaft of humerus** produces **radial nerve palsy.**
63. **Dislocation of the shoulder** would produce **axillary nerve palsy.**
64. **Fractures round the elbow** cause **median nerve palsy.**
65. **Dislocation of the knee** will produce **common peroneal nerve palsy.**
66. **Following fracture pH** rapidly drops to levels in the **acid** range during the **1st 48 hours**.
67. **Longitudinally oriented callus** is laid down by the end of **2nd month.**
68. **pH returns to an alkaline level** higher than normal by the end of the **2nd week.**
69. **Periosteal new bone begins** to proliferate during the **1st 48 hours.**
70. **Rapidly oriented callus** is the main variety by the end of **4th week.**

Chapter three

Traumatic Injury of the Upper Limb

You Should Know

1. **Fracture clavicle is commonest at** the junction of the medial two-thirds and outer/lateral one-third.
2. **Regarding fracture of clavicle,** it is true that:
   - It ensues due to fall on out stretched hand.
   - In children, the type of fracture is greenstick.
   - A figure of eight bandage is used.
   - Distal fragment is depressed.

> ***Note:*** *It is not true that in fractures lateral to the attachment of coracoclavicular ligament displacement is common.*

3. **Most clavicular injuries** result by blows on the point of the shoulder.
4. **Regarding fracture of clavicle:**
   - Healing is rapid.
   - Remodelling even in the adult is very much effective.
   - Pathological fracture may result due to radio necrosis.

> ***Note:*** *Fracture clavicle does not require reduction.*

5. An effective and comfortable **treatment of fracture of the clavicle** is a **sling and analgesics.**
6. In **subluxation of the acromio-clavicular joint, damage** is confined to the acromio-clavicular ligaments.
7. **Diagnostic feature of acromio-clavicular dislocation** includes:
   - The outer end of the clavicle will be prominent while the patient is standing.

- On pushing down the clavicle the contour of the outer end of the clavicle will improve, the elbow being supported from below during this test.
- Displacement of the clavicle seen on radiography.

8. **Various modalities of treatment for cases of acromioclavicular dislocation** may include:
   - Figure of '8' acromioclavicular wiring.
   - Kirschner wires across the joints.
   - Broad arm sling.
   - Coracoclavicular screwing.
9. **Complications of clavicular fractures** may include:
   - Gleno-humeral joint stiffness.
   - A persistent sharp clavicular spike.
   - Extremely rarely non-union.
10. **Regarding scapular fracture:**
    - Usually caused by direct violence.
    - Healing is extremely rapid and excellent.
    - Treatment is by broad arm sling and analgesics.
11. The **appearance of the shoulder** remains normal in **posterior dislocation of the shoulder.**
12. The **appearance of shoulder gets altered** in case of:
    - Anterior dislocation of shoulder.
    - Luxatio in erecta.
    - Subclavicular dislocation of the shoulder.
13. In **dislocation of the shoulder** the usual dislocation of humeral head is sub-coracoid.
14. The commonest **complication of dislocation of the shoulder** is circumflex nerve palsy **(Axillary nerve).**
15. Recognised fracture of **anterior dislocation of the shoulder** includes:
    - Flattening of outer aspect of the shoulder.
    - The arm is held in a position of abduction.
    - Absence of the usual resistance of humeral head on palpating under the edge of the acromion.

- The shoulder is very painful, the patient resents movement.

16. In **posterior dislocation of the shoulder,** the X-ray view most valuable is the axial-lateral view.
17. **Reduction of the dislocated shoulder** is most commonly done by KOCHER's method.
18. **Pathological defects** liable to cause **recurrent anterior dislocation of the shoulder** may include:
    - Rounding of the glenoid margin.
    - Attrition of the anterior shoulder cuff.
    - Flattening of the postero-lateral aspect of the head.
19. **Dislocation of shoulder** downwards with the arm in full abduction results in **luxatio in erecta.**
20. In **recurrent anterior or posterior dislocation of the shoulder** with a joint laxity syndrome "Bone-block repair" is particularly attempted.
21. **"Painful arc syndrome"** may result due to:
    - Subacromial bursitis.
    - Crack fracture of the greater tuberosity.
    - Calcified deposits in the supraspinatus tendon.
    - Crack fracture of the greater tuberosity of humerus.
22. Recognised **feature of painful arc syndrome** includes:
    - Pain appears when the arm is raised to 90°.
    - Pain appears when the arm is lowered from upright position to 120°.
    - Pain is felt in between 60° to 120° of position of arm (abduction).
    - Tenderness below the subacromial area and over the greater tuberosity.
    - X-ray may reveal abnormal subacromial calcification.
23. The optimum time for plaster cast immobilization of a **fusion of a shoulder** is five months.
24. **Patterns of fractures of the neck of humerus** include:
    - Undisplaced crack fracture.
    - Impacted adduction fracture.
    - Undisplaced spiral fracture.
    - Impacted abduction fracture.

25. **Regarding the common type of fractures humeral neck** seen in children:
    - Greenstick fracture without angulation.
    - Greenstick fracture with angulation.
    - Displaced femoral epiphysis.
26. It is true about **fracture of surgical neck of humerus** that:
    - Supinator muscle causes abduction of proximal fragment.
    - It results due to fall on outstretched hand.
    - Fragments are commonly impacted.
    - Distal fragment is adducted or abducted.
27. Regarding **fractures through the anatomical neck of the humerus:**
    - Sometimes seen in fracture dislocation of the shoulder.
    - Caused by a fall on to the point of the shoulder.
    - It is usually a rare phenomenon.
28. Recognised **F/O fractures through the surgical neck of humerus** include:
    - Tenderness over the neck of the humerus.
    - Patient tends to support the arm with the other hand.
    - Obvious deformity in abduction fractures.
    - Gross bruising gravitating down the arm in later stages.
29. Recognised **F/O fracture of upper end of humerus** include:
    - History of trauma.
    - Head is in normal position.
    - Shortening when overlapping is present.
    - Considerable swelling of the shoulder.
30. Regarding **treatment of impacted fracture of the surgical neck of humerus.**
    - The arm is rested in sling.
    - Early shoulder movements should be advised.
    - Some shoulder stiffness may continue for a variable period.
31. Regarding **unimpacted fractures of the surgical neck of humerus:**
    - Majority are abduction injuries.

- Neurological and vascular complications may be there.
- In all cases, reduction should be attempted.
- If closed methods fail, open reduction with internal fixation should be considered.

32. **Pathological fracture from simple bone cyst is common in** the proximal humeral shaft in children.
33. **"A collar and cuff" sling** is useful in treating a case of:
    - Fracture of the greater tuberosity with hairline fracture of humeral neck.
    - Undisplaced segmental fracture of the greater tuberosity of humerus.
    - Comminuted fracture of the greater tuberosity of the humerus.
34. Regarding **fractures of the humeral shaft:**
    - In fractures involving the upper one-third, the proximal fragments tend to be adducted.
    - In fracture involving the middle one-third, the proximal tends to be abducted.
    - Compounding, radial nerve palsy are commonest in middle third fractures.
    - Generally U-slab of POP and collar and cuff sling are sufficient for treatment.
35. **Exploration of the radial nerve in cases of radial nerve palsy** due to humeral fracture shaft should be done if recovery does not commence within 8 weeks.
36. **In fracture of the distal one-third of the shaft of the humerus:**
    - The radial nerve is frequently damaged.
    - Late onset of radial nerve palsy is usually due to involvement of the nerve with callus.
37. Recognised **F/O supracondylar fracture of humerus:**
    - Commonest elbow injury seen in children.
    - The line of fracture is usually oblique from the front of the bone upwards and backwards.
    - Shortening of the arm.
    - Side to side mobility of lower fragment.
    - Brachial artery may be injured.

38. In a **supracondylar fracture of humerus** in a child, admission to hospital is essential following reduction.
39. It is true about the **supracondylar fracture of humerus in a child that**:
    - The distal fragment usually undergoes backwards displacement backward angulation and pronation.
    - The normal equilateral triangular relationship of the olecranon, medial and lateral epicondyle is lost.
    - The fracture line lies just proximal to the bone masses of the trochlea and capitulum.
    - The child is unable to move the elbow.

> ***Note:*** *It is not generally results from a fall on the* ***outstretched hand.***

40. The **supracondylar fracture of humerus** in **children** usually unites within 3 to 4 weeks.
41. **Indication for reduction in cases of supracondylar fracture in children** includes:
    - If there is 50% or less of bone contact.
    - If there is evidence of arterial obstruction.
    - If there is off-ending of the fracture.
    - If there is medial or lateral tilting of 10°or more.
42. Regarding **supracondylar fractures in adults:**
    - Caused by a fall on to the point of the elbow.
    - The fracture line tend to lie a little more proximal than in children.
    - Comminution, obliquity or spiralling are common.
    - 6 to 8 weeks immobilization is usually required.
43. **Volkmann's ischaemic contracture** is most commonly associated with **supracondylar fracture** of the **humerus.**
44. The most important single sign and symptom in suspecting an early Volkmann's ischaemic contracture is **pain.**
45. Regarding **humeral medial epicondylar fracture:**
    - Are usually avulsion injuries.

- Trapping of the medial epicondyle into the elbow joint must be corrected.
- Avulsion may be caused by wrist and finger flexors.
- Avulsion may be caused by medial collateral ligament of the elbow.

46. Regarding **intercondylar Y or T fracture:**
    - Comminution is a problem.
    - Is caused by a fall or blow on the elbow.
    - If there is comminution surgery should not be attempted.
    - In absence of comminution the two main fragments may be opposed with a cross screw.
47. **Posterior dislocation of the elbow** usually result from a fall on the outstretched hand.
48. In **posterior dislocation of the elbow,** the equilateral triangle formed by the olecranon and epicondyle is disturbed.
49. **Forced abduction of the forearm bones** on the humerus may rupture medial collateral ligament.
50. **"Pulled elbow"** results due to sudden pulling on the child's arm.
51. Recognised **F/O the olecranon fracture with intact triceps expansion** includes:
    - Local bruising.
    - Local tenderness and swelling.
    - Clinically no gap will be detectable at the fracture site.
    - Radiologically there will be no separation of the fracture fragments.
52. **Fracture of the olecranon** usually results due to a fall on to the point of the elbow.
53. Recognised **F/O fractures of the radial head** include:
    - Occurs due to a fall on the outstretched hand.
    - Pronation and supination is usually full.
    - Usually bruising and swelling are minimal.
    - The fracture may be comminuted.
54. A **fracture of the radial or ulnar shaft without angulation in a child** requires plaster immobilization for a period of 3 weeks.

55. Regarding **fractures of both forearm bones:**
    - Usually caused by a direct blow.
    - Occasionally caused by torsion of the forearm.
    - When caused by torsion of the forearm the fractures are oblique.
    - When caused by a direct blow the fractures are usually at the same level.
56. The **basic principle in the treatment of fracture of both bones of the forearm** restore normal relationship of radius and ulna.
57. The **"galleazzi fracture dislocation"** consists of fracture of the radius and dislocation of the inferior radioulnar joint.
58. **"Monteggia fracture-dislocation"** is characterized by fracture of the ulna and dislocation of the superior radioulnar joint.
59. Recognised **treatment of galleazzi fracture dislocation** includes:
    - Open reduction and internal fixation.
    - Immobilizations of the arm in an above-elbow plaster.
60. **"Dinner fork"** deformity of wrist is seen in cases of Colles's fracture.
61. In a **Colles' fracture,** the distal fragment is displaced dorsally.
62. **Colles' fracture** occurs in lower end of the radius about ½ to ¾ inch above the articular surface.
63. Regarding **Colles' fracture:**
    - More common in women.
    - Result due to a fall on to the palm of the outstretched hand.
    - The fracture line lies approx 2 cm proximal to the distal articular surface of the radius.
64. **Fracture of radial styloid** was previously known as **Chauffeur's fracture.**
65. **"Smith's fracture"** is the reverse of **Colles' fracture.**
66. **Displacement of the distal radial epiphysis** is confined to **children.**
67. **"Avascular necrosis of the Lunate"** is known as **Kienbock's disease.**

68. The carpal bone most commonly fractured is **scaphoid**.
69. A **transverse fracture of scaphoid** is prone to **avascular necrosis** and usually seen in **young men**.
70. Regarding **carpal navicular fracture**:
    - Prolonged immobilization should be tried.
    - Fragment excision is the last resort.
    - Non-union is common.
    - Pain is over the snuff-box area.
71. The **2nd most common carpal bone to be fractured** is the **lunate.**
72. **Fractured of the scaphoid** is **characterized by**:
    - Tenderness in the anatomical snuff-box.
    - Tenderness on application of pressure over the dorsal aspect of the scaphoid.
    - Tenderness on application of pressure over the palmar aspect of the scaphoid.
73. Recognised **complications of scaphoid fracture** include:
    - Sudeck's atrophy.
    - Non-union.
    - Avascular necrosis.
    - Osteoarthritis.
74. The **carpal bone most commonly dislocated** is the **lunate.**
75. In **arthrodesis of the wrist,** the position of fusion should be **10° to 20° palmar flexion.**
76. **"Mallet finger"** results due to avulsion fracture of the terminal slip of the extensor tendon to the distal phalanx.
77. In **fracture of hand** bones, the hand should be immobilized with position of grasping a base ball.
78. **"Bennett's fracture"** is a fracture dislocation of the **1st metacarpal bone.**
79. **Bennett's fracture** is commonly caused by a blow to the point of the thumb.
80. **Reduction and splintage** are required when three or more metacarpal shafts are fractured.
81. **"Monteggia's fracture dislocation"** may cause injury to:

- Ulnar nerve.
- Median nerve.
- Brachial artery.
- Motor branch of radial nerve.

82. Regarding **fracture of the medial epicondyle of the humerus:**
    - A rotated fragment requires operative reattachment to the epicondyle.
    - It is an avulsion injury.
    - The fragment of bone may be rotated.
83. **Anterior dislocation of the shoulder** may be associated with:
    - Bankart lesion.
    - Damage to the shoulder cuff.
    - Damage to the axillary artery.
    - Fracture of the greater tuberosity.
    - Damage to the brachial plexus.
84. On **radiography, olecranon fracture may be confused for:**
    - Normal bifid olecranon epiphysis.
    - Patella cubiti.
    - Duplication of the normal line due to obliquity of the projection.
    - The normal epiphyseal line.
85. **Internal fixation of the olecranon fragment** may be done by:
    - Acroll olecranon screw.
    - A leg screw.
    - A zuelzer hooked plate and screws.
    - Tension band wiring.
86. **Patterns of fracture of the radial neck** may include:
    - Hairline.
    - Slight tilting.
    - Gross tilting.
    - Complete separation and displacement of the epiphysis of the head.
87. Recognised **complications of Colles's fracture may include:**
    - Mal-union.
    - Sudeck's atrophy.

- Carpal tunnel syndrome.
- Delayed rupture of extensor pollicis longus tendon.
- Persisting stiffness.

88. Regarding "Barton's fracture":
    - A type of Colles' fracture.
    - A type of Smith's fracture.
    - Anterior portion only of the radius is involved.
89. Complications of the **dislocation of the lunate:**
    - Median nerve palsy.
    - Sudeck's atrophy.
    - Avascular necrosis.
    - Secondary osteoarthritis.
90. In **anterior dislocation of the shoulder,** the head of the humerus will be seen lying below coracoid if examined radiologically.
91. **Surgical repairs** for **recurrent anterior dislocation** of the **shoulder** include:
    - The Bankart repair.
    - The Putti platt repair.
92. In **three element fracture dislocation of the shoulder,** the components are:
    - Dislocation of the head of the humerus.
    - Fracture through the surgical neck.
    - Fracture of the greater tuberosity.
93. **Interruption of blood supply to the forearm following "supracondylar fracture** may occur at the time of injury or due to swelling and flexion of the elbow following reduction.
94. **Severely comminuted fracture of the head of radius** should be treated by immediate excision of the radial head.
95. **Colles' fracture** is uncommon below the age **50 years.**
96. In case of **posterior dislocation of the elbow,** the point of the olecranon can be felt to be abnormally posterior to the humoral epicondyles.
97. **Under no circumstances** should the **head of the radius** be **removed in a child.**
98. **Commonest type of shoulder dislocation** is **subcoracoid dislocation** of shoulder.

99. In **acromio-clavicular dislocation,** outer end of the clavicle is prominent.
100. **Lunate dislocation** is given the name of **Kienbock's disease.**
101. **Forced flexion of distal phalanx** is called **mallet finger.**
102. **Fall on dorsum of wrist** produces **Smith fracture.**
103. **Navicular fracture** results when young adults fall with outstretched hand.
104. **Subluxation of the radial head** ensue due to forcible pull of arm.
105. In **trigger finger,** a firm tender nodule is felt in front of the metacarpophalangeal joint.
106. **Mallet finger** results from avulsion or rupture of the extensor digitorum tendon at the base of the terminal phalanx.

> ***Note:*** *Due to unopposed action of the flexor digitorum profundus, the finger gets flexed at the DIP (distal interphalangeal joint).*

107. **Mallet thumb** (Goose neck deformity) results from rupture of the extensor pollicis longus tendon.

> ***Note:*** *It is usually a late complication of Colles' fracture, rheumatoid arthritis etc.*

Chapter four

Traumatic Injury to the Spine

You Should Know

1. The **spinal injury is described as a stable** one if:
   - The neural arch is intact.
   - The articular facets are intact.
   - The posterior ligament complex is intact.
2. **Neurological complications** may ensue in **stable injuries** of the **spine** like:
   - Burst fracture of the spine.
   - Some lateral wedge fractures.
   - Extension injuries of the cervical spine.
3. **Involvement of the cervical spine** should be suspected if the patient:
   - Becomes unconscious after a head injury.
   - Complains of restriction of neck movements following trauma.
   - Complains of neck, occipital or shoulder pain after trauma.
4. If **cervical spine is suspected to be injured,** the 1st move is to keep the head in a neutral position.
5. Recognised **causes of flexion/rotation injuries of the neck** include:
   - Blow on the back of the head from falling objects.
   - Diving in a shallow water.
   - Rapid deceleration in head-on-car accidents.
6. **Stable anterior wedge fracture of the cervical spine** should be treated with a cervical collar for **six weeks.**
7. In a case of **unilateral dislocation of the cervical spine,** the X-ray projection that will confirm the diagnosis is **oblique view.**

8. **Regarding unilateral dislocation of the cervical spine** with a locked facet joint:
   - There is great pain with radiation.
   - Treatment consists of reduction and application of a cervical collar for 6 weeks.
   - If there is any evidence of late subluxation, local cervical fusion should be done.
9. **True dislocation without fracture in spine** can occur only in the cervical region.
10. Evidence of instability in cases of **pure cervical dislocation** may be:
    - Widening of the gap between two spinous processes.
    - Avulsion fracture or fractures.
    - Evidence of forward slip on the flexion lateral X-ray exposure of the spine compared with the extension lateral.
11. In **extension injuries to the cervical spine,** neurological complications are common.
12. In **compression fractures of the cervical spine,** motor pathway to the upper limb is earliest affected.
13. In **compression fractures of the cervical spine** with intact posterior ligament complex, the treatment of choice is cervical traction for **six weeks.**
14. In a case of **compression fracture of the spine,** laminectomy should be considered if:
    - The neurological picture is deteriorating.
    - The cord lesion is incomplete.
    - There is a local block in myelography.
15. It is true about **atlanto-occipital subluxation and dislocation** halo traction after cervical fusion is required.
16. Regarding the **tear of transverse ligaments of the upper cervical region:**
    - There is pain in the neck and the head.
    - There is presence of marked cervical spasm.
    - May be due to rheumatoid arthritis.
    - The gap between the posterior face of the anterior arch and the odontoid is more than 4 mm in adults on lateral view X-ray.

17. **Structures may be confused for odontoid fractures** include:
    - Hypoplasia of the odontoid.
    - Complete absence of the odontoid.
    - Persistent os odontoideum.
18. **Odontoid fracture may result from:**
    - Sudden severe flexion of the neck.
    - Sudden severe extension of the neck.
19. It is true about **spinal fractures** that of the base of odontoid process, the odontoid process is carried forward with the atlas.
20. **Fractures of the thoracic lumbar spine** may result due to:
    - Blow across the back of shoulders.
    - Heavy lifting especially in the middle or advanced aged.
    - Car or motor bike accidents.
    - Fall from a height onto the heels.
21. The **upper limit of wedging of the anterior margin of a thoracic or lumbar vertebra** to get considered as stable is 15°.
22. In **multiple anterior wedging of the thoracic spine,** the lumbar lordosis is increased.
23. The **commonest site of wedge compression of fracture** is lower thoracic upper lumbar.
24. In **retro-spondylolisthesis,** there may be shearing through the:
    - Vertebral body.
    - Pedicles.
    - Discs.
25. **Lumbar transverse process** may be fractured by:
    - Direct trauma.
    - Avulsion.
    - Rotational injury.
26. **Fracture of the transverse process** ensues most commonly in the **lumbar region.**
27. In about **60%** cases, **prolapse of the intervertebral disc** occurs in the **lumbar region.**
28. **Conditions simulating features of ruptured intervertebral disc** include:

- Cases of tuberculosis.
- Cases of osteomyelitis.
- Metastatic tumour.
- Cases of Marie-Strumpell arthritis.

29. **Compression fractures of the cervical spine may result** due to:
    - The head striking the roof in head-on-car accidents.
    - Heavy objects falling on the head.
    - The vertex striking the ground.
30. Recognised **examples of unstable fractures of thoracolumbar spine** may include:
    - Shift of one vertebra relative to another.
    - Wide separation of the vertebral spine at the level of injury.
    - Avulsion fracture of a spinous process.
    - Fracture of the level of the facet joints.
    - Avulsion fracture of the tip of the spinous process.
31. Recognised **conditions predisposed to extension injuries to the cervical neck** include:
    - Klippel-Feil syndrome.
    - Ankylosing spondylitis.
    - Severe rheumatoid arthritis.
32. In **extension injuries to the cervical spine,** the radiographic features may include:
    - Avulsion of anterior longitudinal ligament from its vertebral attachment.
    - Presence of osteophytes.
    - Anterior displacement of pharyngeal shadow.
33. **Fractures of ATLAS** may result from:
    - A fall from a height onto the heels.
    - The head striking the roof of a car in a road traffic accidents.
    - A weight falling on the head.
34. **In a 5th cervical complete cord lesion,** the structures gets paralysed:
    - The arms.
    - The chest.
    - The legs.

35. Recognised **components of "posterior ligament complex" of the spine** include:
    - The supraspinous.
    - The interspinous.
36. **Classification of cervical spine injuries** includes:
    - Flexion injuries.
    - Extension injuries.
    - Flexion and rotational injuries.
    - Compression injuries.
37. **Extension injuries to the cervical spine** is **stable.**
38. The **usual pattern of fractures of the atlas** is **quadripartite.**
39. **Congenital absence of part of the posterior arch of the atlas** may cause confusion for fracture of the posterior arch.
40. **Clay Shoveller's fractures** is a stable fracture injury.
41. **Marked wedging of the anterior margin of a thoracic vertebra** is associated with posterior ligament complex rupture while marked wedging of the posterior margin is possible without rupture of the posterior ligament complex.
42. In **anterior wedge fractures of the lumbar spine,** there is obliteration or reversal of the normal lumbar lordosis.
43. **Prolapse of the disc** is most common in the lumbar region.
44. **Fractures of the pedicles of the axis due to extension injuries with distraction** involve profound neurological involvement.
45. **Fractures of the pedicles of the axis due to extension injuries with compression** involve rarely neurological system.
46. **Sudden severe flexion or extension** involves odontoid fractures.
47. **Sudden muscular contraction** causes Clay Shoveller's fractures.
48. **Transverse ligament lesions** may rupture in rheumatoid arthritis.

49. **Soft tissue injuries of the neck** without fracture due to road accident cause whiplash injuries of the cervical spine.
50. **True dislocations** are commonest in the cervical region.
51. **In the majority of cases, the TB of the vertebra** starts in the **body.**
52. **Spinal shock** indicates transection of spinal cord.
53. The most common cause of **lumbosacral spondylolisthesis** is subchondral bone.
54. The **commonest cause of sciatica** is intervertebral disc prolapse.
55. **Burst fracture of cervical vertebra** is due to vertical compression injury.
56. The **commonest infective lesion of the spine in India is tuberculosis (TB).**
57. The **commonest cause of spinal cord injury in India is fall from a height.**
58. **Severe low back pain** with a sciatic distribution, aggravated by coughing, sneezing and straining, relieved by lying down is most common characteristic of **ruptured intervertebral disc.**
59. The most frequent offending agent in **osteomyelitis of the spine** is—***Staphylococcus aureus.***
60. The **commonest cause of cervicobrachial neuralgia is**—Cervical spondylosis.
61. **Surgical treatment for scoliosis** is indicated when there is:
    - Pain in a scoliotic curve that cannot be controlled by bracing.
    - A unilateral congenital bar in a young child.
    - An increasing curve in a growing child.
    - A severe deformity with asymmetry of the trunk in an adolescent.
62. Scoliosis has been aetiologically associated with:
    - Genetic defect.
    - Pott's disease.
    - Poor posture.
    - Short leg.
63. The **majority of ruptured intervertebral disc** respond successfully to conservative therapy.

64. A **patient has a ruptured disc at level L4, L5.** He typically should show the findings like:
    - Loss of Achilles tendon reflex.
    - Pain over the lower back down leg along lateral calf and dorsum of the foot.
    - Weakness of dorsiflexion of the greater toe.
65. Regarding **Spondylolisthesis**:
    - May be developmental defect.
    - May be the result of a stress fracture.
    - Is a forward slipping of one vertebra upon another usually L5 upon S1.
66. **Diagnosis of spondylolisthesis** is based upon:
    - X-ray evidence of a forward slip of the body of one vertebra upon another.
    - X-ray evidence of a defect in the isthmus portion of the neural arch.
67. **Rupture of the intervertebral disc** most often occurs:
    - In association with 5th lumbar vertebra.
    - Through the annulus fibrosus away from the midline.
68. Recognised **conditions that may resemble the symptoms and physical findings** of a ruptured intervertebral disc include:
    - Metastatic tumour.
    - Tuberculosis.
    - Osteomyelitis.
    - Primary vertebral tumours.
69. **Spondylolisthesis with intact neural arch** is most commonly found between L4 and L5.
70. **Postural scoliosis** may be differentiated from **idiopathic scoliosis** by the fact that postural scoliosis shows curve straightens in forward flexion.
71. **Scoliosis** is most likely to be associated with **cafe-au-lait spots** on skin.
72. **Recognised causes of structural scoliosis** include:
    - Radiation.
    - Neurofibromatosis.
    - Muscular dystrophy.

73. In **congenital scoliosis,** the patterns of curve usually are without pattern.
74. **Narrow lumbar canal syndrome** may cause claudication.
75. The **filum terminale syndrome** is associated with Arnold-Chiari syndrome.
76. Recognised **characteristic of pyogenic infections of the disc space:**
    - Bone scan may show increased uptake in infection.
    - ***Staphylococcus aureus*** is the most common organism.
    - Narrowing of disc space is the first change noted radiologically.
77. Recognised **syndromes caused by a disc space infection** in its early stages include:
    - Meningeal syndrome suggestive of T.B. of acute suppurative meningitis.
    - Abdominal syndrome with suggestion of appendicitis.
    - Hip joint syndrome with signs of a septic joint.
78. **Paraplegia is most often associated with** tuberculosis of the dorsal spine because:
    - Natural tendency to kyphosis in this area.
    - Spinal cord terminates below the level of 1st lumbar vertebra.
    - Spinal canal is smallest in the dorsal area.
    - TB is more common in the dorsal spine.
79. **In a patient with a midline herniated cervical disc:**
    - Equilibrium may be grossly disturbed.
    - Patient rarely complains of pain or stiffness of neck.
80. The **pain similar to that of a ruptured disc** can be produced by pressure on the posterior longitudinal ligament.
81. Regarding **acute osteomyelitis of the sacroiliac joint:**
    - Misdiagnosed as a septic hip.
    - Systemic temperature elevated.

- May present as appendicitis.
- Usually there is history of trauma to the buttocks.

82. Recognised **common C/o patients with Paget's disease** includes:
    - Kyphosis.
    - Backache.
    - Headache.
    - Muscle weakness and fatigue.
83. **The pain of a ruptured cervical disc** may be differentiated from myocardial pain, the latter is usually medial arm pain and the former, lateral arm pain.
84. **In spinal tumour syndrome associated with tuberculosis**, the neurologic sign precede the radiograph of spinal tuberculosis.
85. The **1st sign of pyogenic disc infection** is narrowing of the disc space.
86. **Vertebral plana** initially was believed to be due to aseptic necrosis but recently has been linked to eosinophilic granuloma.
87. A **useful guide indicating completion of vertebral growth** is closure of vertebral ring apophysis.
88. In **Klippel Feil syndrome,** the primary defect is generally believed to be failure of cervical vertebral segmentation.
89. In **Idiopathic scoliosis,** the primary curve is usually thoracic.
90. In a **patient with known tuberculosis of the spine,** the most constant sign of imminent paraplegia due to pressure on the cord is **CLONUS.**
91. **Neurofibromatosis** is associated with:
    - Scoliosis.
    - Skeletal and soft tissue hypertrophy.
    - Congenital pseudoarthrosis.

Note: Neurofibromatosis is not associated with OSTEOCHONDRITIS.

92. **Differentiation of spinal shock** from traumatic shock is often possible in that in the former there is:
    - Alertness.
    - Absence of thirst.
    - A slow strong pulse.
    - Warm, dry skin.
93. **Chordoma** arises from the primitive notochord and has a predilection for the distal and proximal extremes of the axial skeleton.
94. **Most back problems** can be adequately treated with properly fitted support garments.
95. **Priapism** is often a characteristic finding in traumatic lesion of the cervical area of the spinal cord.
96. The **usual treatment of advanced scoliosis in a 14-15 years old patient** is surgical arthrodesis of the affected part of spine because plaster cast cannot maintain correction of scoliosis.
97. In **cases of fracture coccyx severe pain** may occur on walking, sitting or coughing.
98. **Most important single factor in fracture healing** is **immobilization.**
99. **Cervical fracture is treated** by Minerva collars and head traction skull calipers.
100. **Fractures of transverse process of vertebra** occur most commonly in lumbar region.
101. **Dorsal and lumbar fractures** are treated by **hypertension.**
102. **True dislocation** without fracture in spine can occur only in the cervical region.
103. In **children, kyphosis is mainly due to TB** and is rarely congenital.
104. In **adolescence,** adolescent **kyphosis (Scheuermann's disease)** is the commonest cause followed by **T.B.**
105. In **adult,** trauma, osteomalacia, caries spine and Kummell's disease account for most cases of **kyphosis.**
106. In **elderly,** senile kyphosis, senile osteoporosis, neoplastic collapse and Paget's disease are mainly responsible for **kyphosis.**

107. In **case of backache** especially in youngmen, the stress test of spine will feel relief in symptoms in case of ankylosing spondylitis while in pathologies like caries spine, disc prolapse, osteomyelitis and other infection of spine and spinal tumours, etc. patient's symptoms variably aggravated after the test.

108. In **limping,** the patient avoids weight bearing on the affected side as far as possible **(diminished stance phase).**

> ***Note: Limping denotes*** *a painful condition on the affected site.*

109. In **lurching,** the patient **prolongs the stance phase** to improve the stability.

> ***Note: Lurching denotes*** *variable failure of abduction mechanism.*

110. In **Antalgic gait (painful gait),** the patient avoids bearing weight on the affected limb **(reduced stance phase).**

111. **Angle of scoliosis** is measured by **Cobb's method. Ferguson's method** and computer aided assessment of scoliosis.

112. **Investigations for spinal pathology:**

   a. Radiologic investigations

   Plain X-ray < AP / Lat | views

> ***Note: Oblique views*** *are essential to delineate the intervertebral foramen and the facet joints, specially in the cervical region. In lumbar and lumbosacral region, oblique view is used to delineate the integrity of pars interarticularis. In oblique view, this area normally casts a shadow which mimics a* ***Scot terrier's neck.*** *Any defect in pars interarticularis is indicated by a translucent area across the terrier's neck, as if the terrier has been decapitated. This sign is positive in spondylosis and spondylolisthesis.*

b. **Tomography** study (measured depth penetration X-ray) is essential to localise certain less obvious lesions in vertebra, e.g. **osteoid osteoma** and **hemangioma.**
c. **Cine-Radiography:** to know the exclusion of the spinal colum and flow of contrast medium in the subarachnoid space, cine-radiography is of value.
d. **Sonogram** is used to measure **scoliotic curve.**
e. **Contrast radiography** is used to locate any SOL in the spinal canal it utilizes **four** methodology:
   i. Myelographic studies or contrast-dye-radiography
   ii. Air contrast radiography
   iii. Epidurography
   iv. Epidural venography.
f. **Radioactive scanning:** Radiophosphorus or tetracycline, or calcium or strontium are usually used for localizing certain osseous growth or other SOL in the spinal canal.
g. **Discography** is used to assess the prolapse of the disc.
h. **Needle biopsy of vertebral body** is used for:
   - Biochemical studies for **osteoporosis.**
   - Cytological studies for assessing the nature of the **suspected growth.**
i. **Modern imaging techniques.**

> ***Note:*** *These techniques has revolutionized the process of investigating the spinal problem, e.g.*

- CTS (computerised tomography scanning).
- CTS and intrathecal low osmolality contrast media for assessment of pathology such as tumour and dysraphic condition.
- MRI or NMR is extremely sensitive and affords early detection of avascular necrosis, infection, intraspinal disorders (like disc prolapse, and can also distinguish the disc components) cord compression due to trauma and tumour.

> ***Note:*** *It delineates various bony and soft tissue growths without the use of contrast media, differentiation of muscular dysfunction (atrophy, paresis and myopathy).*

- Spinal cord monitoring techniques to record **somato-sensory evoked potential** (SEP) are used mainly during surgical procedure on spine and spinal cord to simultaneously observe any dysfunction of spinal cord, especially while performing corrective surgery for spinal deformity.

Chapter five

Traumatic Injury of the Pelvis and Perineum

You Should Know

1. If only the **superior pubic ramus** is **broken** at one place the period of rest needed is about 2 to 3 weeks.
2. The most common injury due to **fracture of the pelvis** is injury to the **male urethra**.
3. In **fracture of the coccyx** pain occurs on:
   - Defecation.
   - Coughing.
   - Sitting.
   - Walking.
4. **Isolated fractures of the pelvic ring** may result in:
   - Falls from a height
   - Falls on the side.
   - Road traffic accidents.
5. **Posterior dislocation of hip** is most common in hyperextension injury.
6. **Regarding posterior dislocation of hip:**
   - Leg flexed and adducted.
   - Leg is internally rotated.
   - Femoral pulsation is difficult to feel.
   - Greater trochanter is pulled towards anterior superior iliac spine.
7. **Recognized complications of posterior dislocation of hip** include:
   - Avascular necrosis of femoral head.
   - Injury to sciatic nerve.
   - Fracture posterior rim of acetabulum.
8. The commonest dislocation of hip is **posterior.**

9. **Central dislocation of the hip** may result due to:
   - A blow or fall on the side.
   - A fall from a height.
   - A car dashboard injury.
10. **Pelvic injuries** comprise two sets of involvements.
    i. Skeletal framework of pelvis.
    ii. Soft tissues and visceral contents—in the pelvis and around it.
11. The joint in between the sacrum and posterior end of iliac plates are either **amphiarthrodial** (fibro-cartilaginous bridging) or **diarthrodial.**
12. The **normal shape of pelvis** is more or less **signet-shaped.** In **osteomalacia/rickets** under influence of the body weight and thrust of the two femora upwards during locomotion the sacral promontary protrudes antro-inferiorly and the two acetabular floors projects superomedially, giving a **Trefoil** shape of the pelvis.
13. When the **hips** are normal, the pelvis has almost negligible involvement, except for transmitting the weight through the acetabulo-femoral head axis, but in altered situation, the pelvis accommodates disabilities, deformities, and disparities in the length of the lower limbs to a very significant extent. This postural adjustment of the pelvis leads to pelvis obliquity. Pelvic obliquity may be in antro-posterior axis (to accommodate the aforesaid effects in antero-posterior direction) or in lateral axis (to compensate the effects in the side to side axis).
14. In **pelvic injury,** following viscera and soft tissues are likely to be affected depending upon the severity of the fractures.

***Note: The visceras are involved** in following order of frequency.*

i. Urethra and urinary bladder.
ii. Vagina and uterus.
iii. Sciatic nerve.
iv. Rectum and anal canal.
v. Pelvic peritoneum.
vi. Iliac vessels.

15. If one of the bones of the **hemi-pelvis** is fractured, it is not going to affect the integrity of the pelvis in any significant way. This is because the muscles are firmly adapted to the inner and outer pelvic bone plates and act as firm splintage from both sides of the bone.
16. **Pelvis** is common site for inflammatory pathology. Besides the complication following any abdominal and gynecological pathology infection in the form of iliac abscess and psoas abscess are quite common.

> *Note: Being a container with a dependent position, pus and other infected material accumulate at the bottom to present as abscesses (e.g. posas and iliac-psoas abscess in caries spine, infected collection in pouch of Douglas).*

17. Even **major injuries affecting the pelvis** may not be of much significance in males, if visceras and neurovascular bundles are intact. However, in females of childbearing age, any disruption of the normal anatomy or overall shape of pelvis may affect the pregnancy and delivery.
18. In connections with **pelvic examination,** movements at lumbar spine, lumbo-sacral region, hip and sacroiliac region must be tested separately. The movements of the sacro-iliac joints can be tested only by indirect methods i.e. **stress test.**
19. **Stress test are of 4 types:**
    a. Straight leg raising test.
    b. Compression stress test.
    c. Distraction stress test.
    d. Axial rotation stress tests.
       i. Pump handle test.
       ii. Gaenslen's test.
       ii. Laquer's sign.
       iv. Goldthwaite sign.
20. **Straight leg raising test** is also done to test sciatic radiculitis and hip-stability.
21. **Compression stress** test if performed in fractures/dislocation of pelvis, this manoeuvre will elicit pain at the affected side.

22. In **distraction stress test,** similar results and inferences are drawn as in compression stress test.
23. In **pump handle test,** the corresponding side of diseased sacro-iliac joint is tested.
24. **Investigations used in pelvic pathologic states.**

> ***Note:*** *Besides specific investigations indicated for particular pathological conditions, X-ray (in different planes) is an essential investigation for pelvic injuries and pathology.*

The following points must be taken into consideration while taking the radiologic views of pelvis.

a. **Bowel must be cleared** of gases and faecal matter.
b. **Pelvis must be centered** on the X-ray table, i.e. symphysis pubis and umbilicus should be in the same vertical line.
e. The **whole pelvis must be included** in the exposure, rather, inclusion of the lower three lumbar and lower down upto subtrochanteric level is very much helpful in considering the symmetry of the two hemipelvis.
d. In ordering for an X-ray of the pelvis, the clinician must be clear in his mind as to which part he wants to delineate. Antero-posterior X-rays of pelvis inlet, pelvic outlet and sacrum—all require different positioning. One must remember that the pelvis is not placed in a plane horizontal to the long axis of the body, rather, even the fully squared up pelvis is set at an anterior inclination. Therefore, if one wants to have a true antero-posterior exposure for the pelvis, the plate should be placed in contact beneath the pelvis supported on a sandbag and the X-ray beam should be focussed at the centre of the pelvis inlet.

For Sacro-iliac joints

- Place the patient on the X-ray table with a wide sandbag supporting the upper pelvis, i.e. just below the lumbo-sacral areas. The lower limb will be in lithotomy position. The X-ray beam is to be centered on the 3rd sacral body. In this position, the longest zone of the auricle-shaped sacro-iliac joints is traversed by the X-ray beam. Confirmation of correct exposure of the sacro-iliac joints can be had from the fact that the pelvic outlet will project a constricted bean-shaped impression. For exposing the full length of sacrum, place a wide pillow beneath lower lumbar region transversally. Put the patient in wider lithotomy position. The beam is centered to imaginary S3 body.

- Since the sacro-iliac joint is placed obliquely, oblique antero-posterior and postero-anterior views are essential to visualize the joint clearly in its major extent. For oblique postero-anterior view, the patient lies prone. Then the unaffected side of the pelvis is elevated by 30°. The film is centered on the level of the anterior superior iliac spine and the beam is projected centering the midpoint of the film. For oblique antero-posterior view, the patient lies supine and the affected side is elevated by 30°.

> ***Note:*** *For delineating iliac plates, ischial and pubic rami, a plain antero-posterior X-ray exposure is good enough.*

25. **Enumerate Pelvic Injuries**

I. Skeletal injuries

A. Stable fracture (usually due to minor injury)

i. Avulsion (fracture)

e.g.

- Anterior superior iliac spine (sartorius)
- Anterior inferior iliac spine (Rectus femoris)
- Ischial tuberosity (Hamstrings)

ii. Fracture individual pelvic components

- Fracture iliac plates.
- Fracture pubic rami or body.
- Fracture sacrum.
- Fracture coccyx.

iii. Subluxation of the joints.
e.g.
- Pubic symphysis.
- Sacro-iliac joints.
- Sacro-coccygeal joints.

B. Unstable fracture (due to severe injury).
i. Vertical fracture of ilium, pubis and ischium.
ii. Bilateral fracture of ileum, pubis, ischium with various combinations.
iii. Fracture dislocation of pelvis.

II. *Visceral injury.*
- Urethral injury (membranous part of urethra most common).
- Urinary bladder.
- Vagina/uterus.
- Sciatic nerve.
- Rectum and anal canal.
- Pelvic peritoneum with its reflection.
- Iliac vessels.

> ***Note:*** *An extremely rare injury—ipsilateral triple dislocation of pelvic, produces gross instability.*

Triple dislocation means dislocation of hip, sacroiliac joint and pubic symphysis.

26. **Enumerate pelvic disease**

A. Congenital anomalies.
- Undeveloped/underdeveloped pelvis.
- Trefoil pelvis.
- Protrusio acetabuli.
- Ectopia vesicae with deficient pubic symphysis.
- Morphologic alteration as seen in CDH.

B. Inflammatory conditions
- Tuberculous focus in acetabulum and sacro-iliac joints.
- Pyogenic inflammation of iliac plates, specially near about supra-acetabular zone.
- Secondary involvement of pelvic bones following infective conditions of pelvic viscera, iliac abscess, compound injuries and infection abscess.

C. Metabolic and deficiency states
- Rickets
- Osteomalacia (Loosers zone, Trefoil pelvis, protrusio acetabuli)
- Paget's disease.

D. Collagen arthropathy
- Ankylosing spondylitis
- Rheumatoid arthritis.

E. Degenerative conditions
- Degenerative arthrosis of sacro-iliac joint and acetabular margin (hip joints).

F. Tumour or neoplasm

a. Benign
   - Osteochondroma
   - Haemangioma
   - Osteoid osteoma.

b. Malignant
   - Chondrosarcoma
   - Multiple myeloma
   - Secondary carcinomatosis
   - Others (rare).

27. **Pyogenic infection of ilial plate**

    In young children, pyogenic osteomyelitis of lower part of ilium with secondary septic arthritis of hip (and vice versa) is not uncommon.
    - There is systemic and local inflammatory features as in any pyogenic infection.
    - There may be local abscess.
    - Hip movements affected.
    - To **confirm diagnosis,** pus culture and X-ray is mandatory.
    - Treatment according to **culture and sensitivity report.**

28. **TB (tuberculosis) of sacro-iliac joint**
    - The patient is **usually young female** with chronic history of **low backache** and **pain** in the buttock region, specially on changing posture while sleeping, getting up from sitting and vice-versa.
    - Sitting on buttock of affected side is painful, while sitting on the opposite buttock relieves the pain.

- Bending forward with the knee extended is painful (tight hamstrings pulling the sacro-tuberous ligament) whereas bending with the knee flexed (relaxed hamstrings) is painless.
- There is little or no relief by analgesics.
- Localised tenderness, fullness in sacro-iliac joint region.
- May be **cold abscess** in intrapelvic/gluteal region/posterior part of iliac crest.
- Stress test positive.
- Rectal examination demonstrates swelling and tenderness.
- ESR usually not much raised.
- X-ray initially may be non-contributory, later on shows usual changes of tuberculosis.
- Treat the patient with antikoch's drugs.

29. **Ankylosing spondylitis**
    - An HLA-B27 determined disease with familial predisposition.
    - Affects young adults complaining of low backache and morning stiffness, which are relieved after exercise or activity and aggravated after prolonged rest.
    - Male female ratio is 9:1.
    - Deep thrust tenderness over **sacro-iliac regions.**
    - Other associated clinical findings.
    - Pain and stiffness in the dorso-lumbar and both sacro-iliac region which are variably relieved by spinal stress test.
    - More in the morning after getting up from the bed or after getting up from prolonged rest.
    - Patients get comparative relief after daily routine activities walking around or after certain exercises.
    - **Rest aggravates** and **activity relieves the pain and stiffness.**
    - Sometimes bizarre manifestations occur, e.g. pain occurs locally or in generalized all over the body and may be over calf muscles, both heels, shoulder regions, back, and cervical spine.

- Earlier, boarding of back, especially in lower region, later on **poker back** in the advanced cases.
- Restricted spinal movements especially flexion.
- Later on, hip, and still later, shoulder, knee, cervical region, rather all bigger joints to smaller joints (even temporo-mandibular joint) become stiff.
- There may be history of **urethritis**, **uveitis** and **ulcerative colitis.**
- **X-ray**–sacro-iliac joints fusion; bamboo spine due to calcification of collateral ligaments, (periarticular rarefaction, fuzziness across sacroiliac joint, sclerosis of articular margins obliteration of joint line. As pathology advances, trabeculations across the joint).

30. **Osteochondroma**
    - It involves most commonly the **pelvic bones.**
    - Variable knob like irregular, band swelling arising from bone.
    - Symptoms are usually due to pressure effects, cosmetic effects, or when it turns malignant, e.g. chondrosarcoma.
    - X-ray is highly suggestive.
31. **Coccydodynia (coccydynia)**
    - Usually, **overweight ladies** in their **forties**.
    - May or may not be a history of fall on buttock (on the edge of a hard object).
    - **Pain** complained of on sitting on a **hard object**, or **after walking** a long distance, in advanced cases even when passing hard stools.
    - Local tenderness at sacro-coccygeal junction, coccyx, coccygeal tip.
    - **PR examination elicits pain** while finger tip presses posteriorly towards coccyx.
32. **Osteitis pubis**
    - **Painful** condition about the **pubic symphysis** with tendency to spontaneous cure.
    - Exact cause unknown but may follow trauma, usually surgical procedure about the pelvic region, and in woman during pregnancy.
    - **Waddling gait.**

- Lateral compression/distraction tests are positive.
- **Cross leg test positive.**
- Direct pressure elicits **tenderness over pubic symphysis and origin** of **adductor muscles.**
- **Pain** more on abduction of lower limb.
- No local or general signs of inflammation.
- X-ray

  Early stage— No appreciable change.

  Late stage— Pubic bodies look moth eaten, rarefied and gaping, which gradually reossify as normal bony architecture is restored.

33. **Fractures of the pelvis—At a glance**

Introduction: Owing to the **ring structures of the pelvis**, single fractures are often stable and need no treatment other than a few weeks rest. On the other hand, two or more fractures, in the pelvis (with one of the fractures above the level of the hip) renders the ring unstable and this constitute a serious injury, with internal injuries in 25%.

- The force producing the fracture is usually a compression force, often from a traffic accident (60%).

As for example: Fractures of the ilium and pubic ramus (on one or both side), fracture through the sacroiliac joint and a pubic ramus.

- **Malgaigne's fracture:** (20% of all pelvic fractures, 60% unstable ones), disruption of the pelvis anteriorly and posteriorly with displacement of a central fragment containing the hip joint.
- **Acetabular fractures:** common sites; posterior hip or transverse. Two 45° oblique X-rays (± CAT scan) are needed to define injuries exactly.
- **Treatment:** Open reduction and reconstruction of the articular surface to delay the onset of secondary osteoarthritis (OA).

Complications

- Haemorrhage (e.g. from internal iliac artery) check foot pulse, BP, CVP and urine output often. Blood transfusions (BT) may be needed compress early with a pelvic sling.

- **Bladder rupture** may be intraperitoneal or extraperitoneal.
- **Vaginal and rectal perforation:** look for bleeding. Both are rare.
- **Trapping of the sciatic nerve:** there is persistent pain.
- **Rupture of the urethra,** often at the joint of the prostatic and membranous parts in males. The appearance of a drop of blood at the end of the urethra is suggestive. The patient may be unable to pass urine (avoid repeated tries). On rectal examinations (PR examination) the prostate may be elevated out of reach.
- **Treatment:**
  - Relieve pain and replace blood as necessary.
  - Suspend the patient in a pelvic sling promptly.
  - The patient lies supine with the pelvis over the sling's webbing, which exerts upward and medial (compressing) traction via weights and runners suspended above the bed.
  - Traction is also applied to the legs.
  - If rupture of the urethra is possible, insert a suprapubic catheter and urologist may be summoned for expert advice. If only a small volume of urine is found, the reason may be rupture of the bladder.
  - A cystogram may be necessary.

> ***Note: Avoid urethral catheters,** they may make a false passage.*

Chapter six

Traumatic Injury of the Lower Limb

You Should Know

1. Regarding **femoral neck fracture:**
   - It can ensue in young adults due to fatigue.
   - It is common in elderly women.
   - It can occur in young adults following severe violence applied in the long axis of the femur.
2. The **typical deformity in a case of unimpacted fracture** neck of the femur is shortening and external rotation.
3. Regarding **intracapsular fracture of the upper end of the femur** includes:
   - Accompanied by shortening of the leg.
   - Accompanied by external rotation of the leg.
   - Treated by internal fixation.
4. The **femoral head receives its main blood supply** from medullary vessels of the neck of femur.
5. **"Pauwel's angle"** is formed by fracture line of femoral neck with the horizontal plane.
6. **Treatment of choice of early subcapital and midcervical fractures of the neck** in elderly individual is internal fixation.
7. **In cases of intracapsular fractures of the femoral neck, the danger of an impaired blood supply in the proximal fragment increases:**
   - The more proximal is the fracture.
   - The more displaced is the fracture.
   - The more elderly is the patient.
8. In **impacted subcapital fractures,** there is tenderness over the fracture site.

9. **Treatment of choice for unimpacted fracture neck of femur** in patients over the age of 65 years is replacement of the head and neck with a prosthesis.
10. **Fractures of the neck of femur in children** are best treated by open reduction.
11. **Treatment of choice for fractured neck femur** with avascular necrosis of the head in a young individual is internal fixation.
12. **Nonunion in case of fracture neck femur** can be treated by:
    - Subtrochanteric osteotomy in young adults.
    - Replacement of the head by a prosthesis in elderly or if the head is avascular.
    - Insertion of a fibular graft along with renewal of the internal fixation in young adults.
13. **Regarding extracapsular fractures of the neck of the femur:**
    - Nonunion is rare.
    - Avascular necrosis almost unknown.
    - Pertrochanteric type is always comminuted.
    - In pertrochanteric fractures, the leg is more externally rotated.
14. **In fractures in the upper third of the femoral shaft,** the lower fragment is adducted, everted and drawn proximally.
15. A **GALLOWs' Splint** is useful in a case of fracture of the shaft of the femur if the patient is a child below the age of five years.
16. "Y" **shaped fractures of the femoral condyles** may result due to:
    - A fall from a height on to the heels.
    - A direct blow applied to the anterior aspect of the flexed knee.
17. **Disadvantages of conservative treatment for cases of fractures** of the **femoral shaft** may include:
    - Knee stiffness.
    - Prolonged stay in the hospital.
    - Impossible reduction in some cases.
18. In **fractures of the femur,** an intramedullary nail is contraindicated when:

- There is a compound fracture.
- The fracture is 6 inches proximal to the adductor tubercle.
- The fracture is in a child.

19. In **an adult with a fracture of the shaft of the femur,** two liters of blood may be lost without obvious swelling or bruising.
20. In a **transverse supracondylar fracture of the femur,** knee joint is not involved.
21. **Supracondylar fracture of femur** produces backward displacement of distal fragment.
22. **Depending upon the degree of violence a blow on the lateral side of the knee when the patient is bearing weight on the leg can produce:**
    a. Tear of some of the fibres of the medial collateral ligament.
    b. Rupture of the medial collateral ligament.
    c. Peripheral detachment of the medial meniscus besides 'b' above.
    d. Sprain or rupture of one or both cruciate ligaments besides 'c'.
23. **Isolated anterior cruciate rupture occurs** if the knee is forcibly hyperextended.
24. **Isolated posterior cruciate ligament injury** may result due to trauma to the anterior aspect of the flexed knee.
25. **If on flexing the tibia to 90° on the femur excessive forward glide occurs,** it suggests the diagnosis of rupture of the anterior cruciate ligament.
26. **No clearly localised tenderness is demonstrable** if a cruciate ligament is injured.
27. a **"knee snap" heard or felt both during flexion and extension** may be associated with:
    - A cyst of the lateral meniscus.
    - An abnormality of the popliteus tendon.
    - A discoid meniscus.
28. **"Drawer sign"** is diagnostic of injuries of the cruciate ligaments of knee.
29. A **torn meniscus of the knee** occurs when the foot is fixed; the knee is slightly bent and the body is twisted.

30. **Joint line tenderness** is invariable in **meniscus injuries.**
31. The history of sudden **"unlocking"** with a chick and sudden **"locking"** of the knee is suggestive of **meniscus injuries.**
32. The **"cysts of the menisci"** result due to a **myxomatous degeneration.**
33. **Transverse fracture of patella** is usually caused by muscular violence.
34. **Sudden quadriceps contraction** may cause:
    - Avulsion of the tibial tubercle.
    - Rupture of the patellar ligament.
    - Rupture of the quadriceps tendon.
35. The **type of patellar fracture** most difficult to diagnose is **vertical fracture.**
36. **Anatomical conditions predisposing to dislocation of the patella** include:
    - Marked knocked knee.
    - A high patella.
    - A small patella.
    - Usually low lateral femoral condyle.
37. A **comminuted fracture of the patella** should be treated by removal of the patella.
38. Regarding **undisplaced transverse fracture of patella:**
    - Knee joint gets effused.
    - Caused by forcible contraction of quadriceps.
    - Treated by internal fixation.
39. **Osgood, Schlatter's disease is characterized by** recurrent pain, tenderness and swelling over the tibial tubercle.
40. **Active extension is weak or impossible in:**
    - Rupture of the ligamentum patellae.
    - Rupture of the tendinous insertion of the quadriceps muscle into the patella.
41. **Tibia may be fractured** by:
    - Direct blows.
    - Indirect violence.
    - Torsional injuries.
42. Regarding **fracture of the tibial shaft:**
    - Compounding is common.

- In upper tibial fractures, the popliteal artery may be injured.
- May be followed by ischaemia of the distal fragment.

43. **Fracture of the upper end of the fibula** is frequently associated with peroneal nerve palsy.
44. The **tibia** usually takes to **unite radiologically** in **12 weeks.**
45. The **anterior approach to the knee** is an acceptable choice for **ARTHRODESIS.**
46. The **commonest ankle fracture** is external rotation fracture of lateral malleolus.
47. The **ankle joint** is rendered unstable by rupture of the inferior tibio-fibular ligament.
48. The **commonest ankle injuries** are sprains and ruptures of the lateral ligament.
49. **Fracture, without dislocation of the neck of the talus** in an adult may result in viable head and body.
50. Recognised **feature of rupture of the tendo-Achilles includes:**
    - Markedly reduced power of planter flexion.
    - The foot can be dorsiflexed to a greater extent.
    - More common in male in later life.
    - The rupture usually occurs about 3 cm above the insertion of the tendon into the os calcis.
51. Regarding **fracture of the talus:**
    - It results from a fall from a height.
    - Considerable swelling appears rapidly.
    - Infarction of the body of the talus is common.
52. The **most successful treatment for hammer toe** is joint resection.
53. **Plaster boot immobilization** is needed if more than two metatarsals are fractured.
54. **March fracture** is **common** in:
    - Neck of the 2nd metatarsal.
    - Neck of the 3rd metatarsal.
55. Regarding **fractures of the os calcis:**
    - The fracture usually involves the sub-talar joint.
    - Usually caused by falls from a height.
    - If subtalar joint is involved the foot remains stiff irrespective of treatment.

- Degree of displacement varies with the violence.

56. **Important** signs of fracture of the tibial spine include:
    - X-ray finding.
    - Tenderness beneath the ligamentum patellae.
    - Bony block to complete extension of knee.
57. Recognised **feature of congenital discoid lateral semilunar cartilage of knee** includes:
    - Pain on lateral side of the knee.
    - A loud click during the terminal phase of active extension of the knee.
58. **Fracture** of both the tibial and the fibular shafts may occur due to:
    - Road traffic accidents.
    - Torsional injury during ski-ing.
    - Bending during foot-ball play.
59. **Avulsion of the lesser trochanter** occurs due to sudden contraction of the ilio-psoas muscle.
60. **A case of injury to knee** is examined radiologically. Tibia is flexed to 90° on the femur and excessive forward glide is noted. If indicates a rupture of **anterior cruciate ligament.**
61. **In a case of fracture neck femur,** nonunion results. If the patient is elderly and the head is avascular, the treatment of choice is replacement of the head by a prosthesis.
62. The **fracture may be associated with posterior dislocation** includes:
    - Fracture of the femoral neck.
    - Fracture of the posterior lip of the acetabulum.
63. "**McMurray's** manoeuvre" may give positive results in meniscal injury after some days.
64. Recognised **components of the extensor apparatus of the knee** include:
    - The quadriceps muscle.
    - The tendinous insertion of the quadriceps muscle into the patella.
    - The patella retinaculae.
    - The patella.
    - The ligamentum patellae.

- The insertion of the ligamentum patellae into the tibial tubercle.

65. **Types of extracapsular fractures of the proximal femur** include:
    - Basal cervical.
    - Pertrochanteric.
66. **"Thomas' splint" is used for** fracture of the shaft of the femur.
67. Recognised **types of tear of the meniscus** include:
    - Anterior horn tear.
    - Posterior horn tear.
    - Bucket handle tear.
68. In **cases of posterior dislocation of hip,** the leg is flexed adducted and internally rotated.
69. In **cases of anterior dislocation of hip,** limb is in a position of flexion, abduction and external rotation.
70. The **Achillis tendon** is the commonest tendon in numan body to rupture.
71. **Avulsion of the styloid process of the 5th metatarsal** occurs due to contraction of the peroneus brevis during forced inversion of the foot.
72. **Shortening and external rotation** is seen in **fracture neck femur.**
73. Flexion, adduction and internal rotation is seen in **posterior dislocation of the hip.**
74. Abduction and external rotation is seen in **anterior dislocation of the hip.**
75. **Central dislocation of the hip** involves fracture of acetabulum.
76. **Sudden muscle contraction of erector spinae** causes avulsion fracture of posterior iliac spine.
77. **Sudden muscular contraction of rectus femoris may** cause avulsion of anterior inferior iliac spine.
78. **Sudden muscle contraction of sartorius** may cause avulsion fracture of anterior superior iliac spine.
79. **Sudden muscular contraction of hamstrings** may cause avulsion fractures of ischial tuberosity.

80. **Sudden muscular contraction of abdominal muscles** may cause avulsion fracture of abdominal muscles.
81. **Relatively minor violence on the lateral aspect of the knee** may cause rupture of some fibres of the medial collateral ligament.
82. **A frontseat passenger in a motor car** is thrown violently forward against the dash board may cause **posterior cruciate rupture.**
83. The **knee joint** is forcibly hyperextended in cases of isolated anterior cruciate rupture.
84. **When knee is struck on its medial side** it will cause injury to the lateral collateral ligament.
85. **Second degree Pott's fracture** is also called **Bimalleolar fracture.**
86. In **first degree Pott's fracture**, only one malleolus is involved.
87. **Bimalleolar fracture** of a fracture of the posterior part of the inferior articular surface of the tibia is designated as **third degree Pott's fracture.**

Chapter seven

Diseases of Bones and Joints or Cold Orthopaedics

You Should Know

1. **Treatment of choice for solitary bone cyst** is curettage with bone grafting.
2. **Blotchy calcification on X-ray** is present in→chondrosarcoma.
3. **"Barlow's sign"** is diagnostic of congenital dislocation of hip (CDH).
4. **Haemangiomas of bones** are most often found in the vertebrae.
5. **Osteochondritis of lunate** is called Keinbock's disease.
6. **Osteochondritis** that presents at the earliest age (4 to 10 years) is Perthes' disease.
7. Tumour that most often cause a solitary metastasis is **kidney**.
8. **Looser's zone** or **pseudofractures** are characteristic of **osteomalacia.**
9. Most common cause of **Pes cavus** is→**Idiopathic**.
10. Muscles commonly involved in **Volkmann's ischaemic contracture** include:
    - Pronator quadratus.
    - Flexor pollicis longus.
    - Flexor digitorum profundus.
11. **Anterior scalloping of vertebral bodies** is present in:
    - Aortic aneurysm.
    - Tuberculous spondylitis.
    - Down's syndrome.
12. **Commonest site of pigmented villonodular synovitis** is→**knee**.

13. **Finkelstein's test** is positive in **de-Quervain's tenosynovitis.**
14. **Tenosynovial infection of the index finger** most likely would extend first into→**Thenar space.**
15. **Phalen's test** is positive in→**carpal tunnel syndrome.**
16. **Double structural scoliotic curves** are typically seen in→**Marfan's syndrome.**
17. **Onion-peel appearance** on radiography is seen in **Ewing's sarcoma.**
18. Commonest cause of **genu varum is→Rickets.**
19. **Commonest primary malignant bone tumour** is **osteogenic sarcoma.**
20. **Genu varum is seen in** Rickets, Blount's disease and Paget's disease.
21. **"Bamboo spine"** results from→Ankylosing spondylitis.
22. Joint fused in **"triple arthrodesis"** includes Talocalcaneal, talonavicular, and calcaneocuboid.
23. **Pseudoarthrosis** following triple arthrodesis mostly seen in talonavicular joint.
24. **Bilaterally symmetrical sacroilitis** is seen in ankylosing spondylitis, psoriatic arthropathy and hyperparathyroidism.
25. **"Spina ventosa"** results from→Tuberculosis.
26. **"Gaenslen's operation"** is done for sacroiliac subluxation.
27. **Majority of ruptured intervertebral discs respond to**→conservative therapy.
28. Carcinoma most likely to develop in chronic osteomyelitis is **squamous cell C_A.**
29. The most important single sign in **impending Volkmann's ischaemic contracture** is→ **Stretch pain.**
30. The nerve that has autonomous sensory zone enabling functional evaluation is→**Ulnar nerve.**
31. In **acute haematogenous osteomyelitis,** the earliest X-ray changes in bone are seen in→**Ten days.**
32. A **graft of tissue** (bone) into a dissimilar tissue is known as **Heterotopic.**

33. **"Melon seed bodies"** are characteristic of **tubercular tenosynovitis (T.B.).**
34. **Froment's sign** is diagnostic of **ulnar nerve palsy.**
35. **Ewing's tumour** is diaphyseal.
36. In **patient's with sickle cell anaemia,** osteomyelitis usually results from→**Salmonella typhi.**
37. In **rheumatoid arthritis,** there is primarily involvement of synovial membrane.
38. **Codman's tumour** is **chondroblastoma.**
39. **Lamina dura of teeth** is **not seen in** primary hyperparathyroidism, Cushing's syndrome and Paget's disease.
40. **Triple arthrodesis** for **severe deformities of foot** is done when the patient is atleast **10 years** old.
41. **Finding of phosphoethanolamine** in urine is pathognomic of **hypophosphatasic rickets.**
42. **Osteoclastoma** present as expansile osteolytic area in the epiphysis and metaphysis.
43. **Sudden attack of** acute pain in great toe with redness is due to **gout.**
44. **Corticomedullary differentiation** is absent in **osteopetrosis.**
45. **Ring type of sequestrum** is present in lower part of bone after **amputation.**
46. The **treatment of osteoclastoma** of the upper end of the humerus is excision followed by fibular graft.
47. **Van der Hoove's syndrome** consists of otosclerosis, osteogenesis imperfecta and blue sclera.
48. **Hip disarticulation** provides best treatment for fibrosarcoma of mid thigh.
49. In **Multiple exostosis**, treatment is required because of mechanical obstruction of joints.
50. **Treatment of choice in psoriatic arthropathy is** Methotrexate.
51. **Froment's sign** is positive due to the **paralysis** of **adductor pollicis.**

52. **Head of femur** between the ages of **4 to 9 years** gets its blood supply from **lateral epiphyseal vessel.**
53. In the **management of active rickets,** vitamin D and calcium should be given both pre- and post-surgery.
54. **Earliest bone metastasis** can be detected by **Radio-isotope bone scan.**
55. **"Tumbling bricks" appearance** in an X-ray of the spine is seen in **Neurosyphilis.**
56. In **functional position of hand,** meta-carpophalangeal joints are held at flexion of **60°.**
57. **Cubitus valgus** is usually seen in fracture of lateral condyle of humerus.
58. Commonest C/P of osteoporosis is **chronic backache.**
59. **Meralgia paraesthetica** is due to compression of lateral cutaneous nerve of thigh.
60. In **Rheumatoid arthritis,** serum complement level is reduced.
61. Ortolani's test is done for CDH (cong. dislocation of hip).
62. **Rheumatoid arthritis** is an inflammatory arthritis.
63. **Tom-Smith arthritis** involves head of femur.
64. **Chondroma** is a malignant tumour.
65. **Dupuytren's contracture** is more common in **Alcoholics.**
66. **Osteoblastic type of secondaries** are produced by **C_A prostate.**
67. **Treatment of choice for Paget's disease** of bones **is calcitonin.**
68. **Earliest evidence of healing in rickets** is provided by radiological examination of growing end of bones.
69. **Drug used in treatment of osteoporosis** is progesterone, oestrogen and anabolic steroid.
70. The commonest cause of **septic arthritis** in young adults is gonococcal arthritis.
71. **Osteochondritis dessicans** commonly involves **knee joint.**

72. **Painless effusion in joints in congenital syphilis** is called **Charcot's joints.**
73. Commonest skeletal abnormality seen in **rickets** is **Genu valgum.**
74. **Medial semilunar cartilage** is commonly damaged in knee joint because attached to tibial collateral ligament.
75. In **ankylosing spondylitis,** radiological changes are first seen in sacro-iliac joints.
76. **Osgood-Schlatter disease** is epiphysitis of the **tibial tubercle.**
77. **Epiphyseal enlargement** is seen in **hemophilia.**
78. Bone secondaries from **breast carcinomas are** osteolytic.
79. Normal atlantoaxial diameter in an adult is **2.5 mm.**
80. **Triple deformity of knee** is seen in **tuberculosis.**
81. **Bone erosion** is seen in gout, rheumatoid arthritis, osteoarthritis and psoriasis.

> ***Note:*** *Bone erosion does not occur in SLE.*

82. **Alkaline phosphatase is elevated in** Paget's disease, osteomalacia, multiple myeloma.

> ***Note:*** *Alkaline phosphatase is not elevated in osteoporosis.*

83. **Pain in thigh more at night**, relieved by aspirin is seen in osteoid osteoma.
84. **Bone sclerosis** is seen in fluorosis, osteopetrosis and second axis from prostate.
85. **Bone tumour metastasizing to bone** is Ewing's sarcoma.
86. **Osteoclastoma is common in age group** of 20 to 40 years.
87. **Syme's amputation** is contraindicated in **diabetic foot.**
88. **Vertical striations** on vertebral bodies are seen in **haemangioma.**
89. **Soft tissue calcification** occurs in hyperparathyroidism, scleroderma and hypervitaminosis 'D'

> ***Note:*** *It is not seen in hyperthyroidism.*

90. **Tom Smith arthritis** differs from other arthritis in that mobility is retained.
91. The **EMG change characteristic of denervated muscle** is fibrillation potentials.
92. In **spinal muscular atrophy,** the site of lesion is anterior horn cell.
93. **Madelung's deformity** involves **wrist.**
94. **Keinbock's sign** is positive in injury to scaphoid.
95. **Septic arthritis of hip in infants** is referred to as **Tom Smith arthritis.**
96. **Diaphyseal achalasia** is seen with **multiple exostosis.**
97. **Kernige's sign** is tested by extension of knee, flexion of hip.
98. **Reactive arthritis** is caused by **Shigella**.
99. **Caries sicca** is tuberculosis involvement of **spine**.
100. Multiple punched out lesion in skull is seen in **Multiple myeloma.**
101. **Sunray appearance of X-ray** is seen in **osteogenic sarcoma.**
102. **Phocomelia** is gross reduction in proximal part of extremity.
103. **Osteoporosis** is seen in Cushing's syndrome, thyrotoxicosis, and long-term heparin therapy.

> *Note: It is not seen in hypoparathyroidism.*

104. **Commonest cause of kyphosis** in young adult males is→Ankylosing spondylitis.
105. **Longitudinal growth of bone** is by epiphyseal plate.
106. In **disc prolapse of C5-6** the nerve root pressed is **C6.**
107. **Remodelling** is **not seen** in **rotational deformity**.
108. **Pseudoarthrosis of tibia** is treated by internal fixation and bone grafting.
109. **Periarticular erosion** are seen in gout, osteoarthritis and rheumatoid arthritis.
110. **Carpal tunnel syndrome** is seen in myxedema, pregnancy and Colles' fracture.
111. Hypermobile flat foot is found in old age, Marfan's syndrome, Ehler-Danlos syndrome.

112. In **ankylosing spondylitis,** the joints involved are sacroilaic shoulder and hip and knee joints.

> *Note: Hands and wrist joint are not involved in ankylsoing spondylitis.*

113. **Pseudoarthrosis of tibia** is most commonly associated with neurofibromatosis.
114. **Benign neoplasm of bone** alone presents with pain is→osteoid osteoma.
115. In **osteoarthritis (OA),** there is preservation of bone density.
116. **Romanus lesion** is characteristic of ankylosing spondylitis.
117. **"Wandering acetabulum"** is seen in **tuberculosis of hip.**
118. **Pillow splint** used in gradually abducting an infant's hip in CDH is **Frejka splint**.
119. **Yergason's test** is associated with **bicipital tendinitis.**
120. **"Aird's test"** is done for **Malingener's back pain.**
121. **"Erlenmayer flask appearance" of femur** is seen in→**Gaucher disease.**
122. **Paraplegia** is more common in TB of upper dorsal spine because cord canal ratio is low.
123. **Large epiphysis with early epiphyseal closure** is seen **in juvenile chronic arthritis.**
124. **Osteosclerosis** with ligamentous calcification is seen in→**Fluorosis**.
125. **"Trigger finger"** is usually associated with rheumatoid tenosynovitis.
126. **"Adson's test"** is useful in diagnosis of→Cervical rib.
127. **Ossification** begins in foetus in **5th week of IUL.**
128. The enzyme found in the osteoclast but not in osteoblast is **acid phosphatase**.
129. **Viscosity of synovial fluid** is dependent on the concentration of **hyaluronic acid.**
130. **"Hook sign"** is positive in suppurative flexor tenosynovitis.
131. **De Quervain's disease** classically affects the extensor pollicis brevis and abductor pollicis longus.

Chapter eight

Congenital and Developmental Diseases of Bones

You Should Know

1. **"Von Rosen"** or **"Barlow's sign"** is found in cases of CDH (Congenital dislocation of hip).
2. **Bilateral congenital dislocated hips are associated** with:
   - Waddling gait.
   - Positive Trendelenburg sign.
   - Positive Allis sign.
   - Shenton's line defect.
3. Regarding **congenital dislocation of hip (CDH):**
   - The condition is more common in girls.
   - Breech malposition of the foetus is an important aetiologic factor.
   - The hip is either dislocated or dislocatable at birth.
   - Conventional clinical exam's of the hip is normal at birth.
   - Presence of waddling gait in late bilateral cases.
4. **Radiologic features of CDH in a child of two years include:**
   - Shallow acetabulum.
   - A break in Shenton's line.
   - Small capital femoral epiphysis.
   - Lateral and upward displacement of the epiphysis of the femoral head.
5. The **upper age limit for treating a case of bilateral congenital dislocation of hips** is →**Four years.**
6. The **upper age limit for treating a case of unilateral CDH** is **7 years.**

7. **"Blount's disease"** is characterized by progressive genu varum.
8. **Congenital pseudoarthrosis of the tibia** usually starts with anterior bowing of the tibia.
9. **Abnormalities of the foot and ankle** are associated with postero-medial bowing of the tibia.
10. The **most common variety of congenital club foot** is congenital talipes equino-varus.
11. **Recognised feature of congenital talipes equinovarus** includes:
    - Present since birth.
    - Usually bilateral.
    - Histologically normal skin, subcutaneous tissues and muscles.
    - Presence of a transverse crease across the sole of the medial side.
12. **Regarding Talipes equinovarus:**
    - Make up 75% of congenital foot anomalies.
    - There is no bone deformity at birth only disturbed relationship.
    - A congenital condition mainly affecting male babies.
    - Cause is failure to rotate from atal position.
    - The medial and plantar soft tissues and calf muscles are contracted.
13. **Recognised feature of Talipes equinovarus includes:**
    - Inversion of the os calcis.
    - Plantar flexion of all the bone of the forefoot including the talus.
    - Hypoplastic but histologically normal calf muscles.
    - Adaptive shortening of the skin on the concave side of the curve.
14. **To detect minor degree of talipes equinovarus at birth,** there is inability to dorsiflex the foot so as to touch the anterior.
15. **In talipes calcaneal valgus,** the foot is dorsiflexed and everted.
16. The **most common cause of bunion deformity** is **metatarsus primus varus.**

17. A **clinical condition in which the whole shoulder girdle is higher on the affected side** than on the normal side is SPRENGEL'S shoulder.
18. The **most common coalition in tarsal coalition** is medial talocalcaneal bar.
19. Regarding **congenital vertical talus** the sole is convex downwards.
20. **Congenital absence of the fibula is associated with:**
    - Forward bowing of the tibia.
    - An equino-valgus deformity.
    - Absence of the 5th toe.
21. **Recognised feature of cleidocranial dysostosis may include:**
    - The patient can bring his shoulders together in front of the chest.
    - Large head and a relatively small face.
    - The clavicles are almost completely absent.
    - Development of membranous bone is faulty.
22. **Cleidocranial dysostosis may exhibit:**
    - Brachycephaly.
    - Large foramen magnum.
    - Complete absence of clavicles.
    - Coxa vara of femur.
23. **Recognised feature of congenital radioulnar synostosis includes:**
    - May be unilateral or bilateral.
    - Foramen in a pronated position.
    - Proximal radius may be absent.
    - Proximal radius may be present but dislocated.
24. **Abnormality in growth of the distal radial epiphysis occurs in** Madelung's deformity.
25. In **congenital dislocation of the radial head,** the radial head may be displaced posteriorly, anteriorly and laterally.
26. Regarding **congenital pseudoarthrosis of the clavicle** it is confined to females.
27. **Myelodysplasia** is least common in thoracic region.
28. In **myelodysplasia,** posterior elements of the vertebra are absent.

29. **Hemivertebrae** are responsible for→ SCOLIOSIS.
30. **Recognised features of osteogenesis imperfecta may include:**
    - Multiple fracture.
    - Bone osteoporosis.
    - Blue sclerotics.
    - Deafness.
31. **Multiple exostosis** is characterised by variable number of exostoses developing in the metaphyseal region of the long bones.
32. **Dyschondroplasia is characterised by** multiple euchondromata of the fingers and toes.
33. **Malignant change develops in** about **1%** of congenital chondromas.
34. **Recognised features of Albers-Schonberg disease (Marble bones) include:**
    - The bone is hard.
    - Fractures are common.
    - For practical purposes medullary canal is absent.
    - A rare familial disease.
    - On X-ray, bones appear excessively dense and structureless.
35. **Recognised features of Nail-Patella syndrome may include:**
    - Small patellae.
    - Hypoplastic or absent nails.
    - Lateral subluxation of the radial head.
    - Bony excrescences on the lateral aspect of the ileum.
36. **Morquio-Brailsford's disease (Chondro-osteodystrophy)** is characterised by:
    - Tri-radiate pelvis.
    - Typical "tonguing" of the vertebral bodies on X-ray.
    - Consanguinity is an important aetiological factor.
    - Produced by a recessive gene.
37. In **schondroplasia,** the patient is **dwarfed.**
38. **Dwarfism** may be caused by:

- Gargoylism.
- Chondro-osteodystrophy.
- Achondroplsia.
- Epiphyseal dysplasias.

39. **Genu-valgum** is the condition of **knock-knee.**
40. **Cubitus varus** is the condition of **adduction of forearm.**
41. A combination of **meningomyelocele and hydrocephalus** is invariably a sign of ARNOLD-CHIARI deformity.
42. **Spina bifida along with meningomyelocele may cause:**
    - Paralytic deformities of foot.
    - Incontinence of urine.
    - Incontinence of faeces.
    - Trophic ulcers.
43. **Regarding spina bifida occulta:**
    - Occurs due to failure of the neural arches to unite.
    - Foot-drop, nocturnal enuresis may occur in later life.
    - A fibrous band connects the skin to the spina theca.
    - Many cases are symptomless.
44. **PHOCOMELIA** is most commonly due to **Thalidomide.**
45. Eliciting a click from the hip in cases of CDH is known as **Barlow's sign.**
46. **Recognised feature of genu varum includes:**
    - May be caused by an epiphyseal dysplasia.
    - Is commonly seen in infants and mild cases are normal.
    - Also called bow leg or bandy leg.
    - Requires surgery if at about age four the knees are two inches apart when the medial malleoli are together.
    - Is not usually necessary as spontaneous correction occurs.
47. **Macewen's osteotomy** is classically performed for **Genu Valgum.**

48. **Recognised feature of "Nail-Patella" syndrome** includes:
    - Small patellae.
    - Radial head may subluxate laterally.
    - Bony excrescences may develop on the lateral aspect of the ilium.
49. **Regarding spondylolisthesis:**
    - May be the result of a stress fracture.
    - May be a developmental defect.
    - Is a forward slipping of one vertebrae upon another usually L5 upon S-1.
50. **Diagnostic feature of CDH (unilateral) at one year of age includes:**
    - Symmetrical skin creases in the groin and around the buttocks.
    - Positive Trendelenberg's sign.
51. **Regarding Ollier's disease (Chondromatosis):**
    - Involved bones are often expanded by the tumour.
    - Ossification of the cartilage at the epiphyseal palate is faulty.
    - Radiologically lytic lesion expanding the bone is evident.
52. **Fusion of cervical vertebrae** is seen in **Klippel-Feil syndrome.**
53. A **positive "Trendelenberg's sign"** is **produced by:**
    - Congenital dislocation of hip (CDH).
    - Paralysis of the abductors of the hip.
    - Fracture of the neck of femur.
54. In **bilateral CDH,** there is **waddling** gait.
55. **Von Rosen splint** is useful for treating a case of **CDH** in the **newborn infant.**
56. In **internal tibial torsion,** the lateral malleolus is parallel or at times, anterior to the medial malleolus.
57. **Genu varum** is **normally present** in the **newborn.**
58. **Genu valgum** is **normally present** between **three and 10 years of age.**
59. The **most common site for myelomeningocele** is the **lumbar region.**

60. **Congenital anterior bowing of the tibia** generally progresses to a pathological fracture and congenital pseudoarthrosis of the tibia.
61. **Flat foot** with full range of movement supple **pes planus.**
62. Commonest type of congenital club foot is **Talipes-equino-varus.**
63. First metatarsal in a varus position, others in a normal position is **metatarsus primus coalition.**
64. When all the metatarsal in a varus position→**Metatarsus varus.**
65. Fusion of one or more tarsal bones→**Tarsal coalition.**
66. **"Leri's disease"** is related to **candle bones.**
67. **Apert's syndrome** is associated with **Acrocephalo-syndactyly.**
68. **Marphan's syndrome** has **spider finger (Arachnodactyly).**
69. **Osteopathia striata** exhibits **striped bones.**
70. **Osteo-poikilosis** shows **spotted bones.**

Chapter nine

Inflammatory and Degenerative Diseases of Bones and Joints

You Should Know

1. The most frequent **site of predilection** for **acute osteomyelitis** is **metaphysis of the long bones.**
2. The usual causative organism of acute osteomyelitis is ***Staphylococcus aureus.***
3. In **haematogenous osteomyelitis,** the earliest X-ray changes in bone may be seen in **10 days.**
4. The most common causative organism of **osteomyelitis** in cases of **sickle cell anaemia** patient is ***Salmonella* organism.**
5. The most striking feature of **haematogenous osteomyelitis** occurring in infants is the **low fever** and **lack of toxicity.**
6. **Sequestrum** in acute osteomyelitis of an adult usually separates within 3 months.
7. The **earliest radiographic evidence of osteomyelitis** is not evident until **10 to 14 days** from the onset of the infection.
8. The **bone infarct** in acute osteomyelitis is known as **sequestrum.**
9. A **dead piece of bone** is called as **sequestrum.**
10. On **radiography,** a long bone shows a circular cavity surrounded by a zone of sclerosis, the most probable diagnosis is→**Brodie's abscess.**
11. **Regarding Brodie's abscess:**
    - It is a cavity surrounded by densely sclerosed bone.
    - Small sequestra are usually presents inside the cavity.
    - It resemble bone cyst, but sclerosis is absent.

- It is a type of chronic osteomyelitis.
- It is usually seen in metaphyseal region.

12. **Brodie's abscess** in a long bone is seen in cases of **chronic osteomyelitis.**
13. The joints specifically **predisposed to septic arthritis** secondary to osteomyelitis is **hip and knee joints.**
14. **Tuberculosis of the spine** is thought to originate from the muscle attachments.
15. The earliest and most consistent sign of **spinal tuberculosis** in a child is **pain on sudden motion.**
16. **Paraplegia** occurs most commonly in **spinal tuberculosis** when involvement occurs in the **high thoracic spine.**
17. The definite treatment of spinal TB is usually **spinal fusion.**
18. **Swelling of tuberculosis knee joint** is due to **thickening of synovial membrane.**
19. Most frequent **osteoarticular TB** is seen in **spine.**
20. **"Melon-seed" bodies** are found in cases of **tuberculous tenosynovitis.**
21. **Bony ankylosis may follow:**
    - Osteoarthritis
    - Pyogenic arthritis
    - Tuberculous arthritis
22. The earliest and most constant radiographic finding of spinal tuberculosis is **narrowing of intervertebral disc.**
23. **Congenital syphilis** affecting bone characteristically exhibits:
    - Serous synovitis
    - Sabre shin (tibia)
    - Mainly epiphyseal lesion
    - Inhibition of osteoid production.
24. In **actionmycotic osteomyelitis,** the antibiotic of choice is→Penicillin.
25. The DOC for **coccidioidomycosis osteomyelitis** is Amphotericin-'B'.
26. In **sarcoidosis,** serum globulin is usually elevated.
27. **Recognised feature of rheumatoid arthritis includes:**

- The disease is usually polyarticular.
- The small joints of the hand and feet are usually 1st affected.
- Morning stiffness of joints.
- Subcutaneous nodules usually appear on extensor surface of upper arm.
- Amyloidosis may complicate the disease.

28. **In RA (Rheumatoid arthritis)**, the most common extensor tendon to rupture is→**Extensor pollicis brevis.**
29. **The pathology of rheumatoid arthritis (RA) includes:**
    - Joints do ankylose.
    - Vasculitis.
    - Joints breaking down and becoming unstable.
    - Degeneration of all tissues containing collagen.
    - Joint synovium showing lymphoid foci rather than a generalised inflammation.
30. The **"Swan** neck" deformity seen in cases of RA results due to contracture of intrinsic muscles of the hand.
31. The **earliest radiologic feature of rheumatoid arthritis** is narrowing of the joint space.
32. **Recognised feature of ankylosing spondylitis includes:**
    - Starts in early adult life.
    - Central joints of the body are involved.
    - Calcification followed by ossification of the ligaments and joint capsules.
33. **The joints most commonly affected in ankylosing spondylitis is**→sacro-iliac joint.
34. **"Bamboo spine"** results due to ankylosing spondylitis.
35. **Regarding osteoarthritis (OA):**
    - Uncommon in childhood.
    - May affect only one joint.
    - Its greatest disability is when the hip joints are affected.
    - Is associated with loss of weight-bearing cartilage as an early change.

36. **Osteoarthrosis (OA) may follow:**
    - Rheumatoid arthritis.
    - Septic arthritis.
    - Tuberculous arthritis.
    - Injury to a joint.
37. **Osteophytes are characteristic feature of** →osteoarthritis (OA).
38. The **earliest pathological feature of osteo-arthrosis is**→Fibrillation of the cartilage.
39. **Recognised feature of osteoarthrosis includes:**
    - Pain at night.
    - Increasing stiffness of the joint.
    - A limp, if joints of the lower limb are involved.
40. The **earliest X-ray picture of OA** is **narrowing of joint space.**
41. **Chondromalacia patellae** results due to **osteoarthrosis.**
42. **Regarding cervical spondylosis:**
    - It is a degenerative disc disease.
    - Osteophyte may cause radicular symptoms.
    - Cervical traction may alleviate the symptoms
    - Surgical removal of the osteophytes may be needed.
43. **Areas of** maximum tenderness in cases of supraspinatus tendinitis is over the acromian.
44. **Rotator cuff** about the shoulder consists of:
    - Subscapularis tendon.
    - Infraspinatus tendon.
    - Supraspinatus tendon.
    - Teres minor muscle tendon.
45. The **most commonly torn tendon in cases of rotator cuff tear** is SUPRASPINATUS tendon.
46. **Regarding the bicipital tendon rupture:**
    - Common in older individuals.
    - The patient usually present with a mass in the anterior arm.
    - Muscle belly of the biceps is located distally.
    - In young individual, surgical correction is required.
47. The **treatment of choice for Frozen shoulder** is active exercises eliminating gravity.

48. **Tennis elbow is a tendinitis** of the origin of the **common extensor and supinator muscles** from the lateral epicondyle.
49. Trigger finger or **trigger thumb** results due to **tendinitis** of **flexor tendons.**
50. **De-Quervain's disease** results due to inflammation of the extensor pollices longus and the abudctor brevis tendon.
51. **Rheumatoid factor** may be found in syphilis, SLE and leprosy (Hansen's disease).
52. **Dupuytren's contracture** usually affects initially the **little finger.**
53. **Recognised feature of supraspinatus tendonitis includes:**
    - Localised tenderness over the insertion of supraspinatus tendon.
    - Pain in the shoulder especially on abduction and rotation.
    - Rapid onset of shoulder stiffness.
    - Causes "Painful arc syndrome."
54. **"Carpal tunnel syndrome"** may result due to rheumatoid arthritis, pregnancy and myxedema.
55. **Regarding ganglia:**
    - Localised tense cystic swellings.
    - Often communicates with a tendon sheath or the capsule of a joint.
    - Their origin is uncertain.
56. **Recognised feature of acute osteomyelitis in adults includes:**
    - No significant bony change for 2 to 4 weeks.
    - Course is milder when compared to that in children.
    - Starts analyze as there is no metaphysis.
    - Septic arthritis is a frequent complication.
57. **Regarding ankylosing spondylitis:**
    - Can be partly diagnosed by tissue typing (HLA-B27).
    - Tends to begin in the sacro-iliac joints.
    - Is a variant of rheumatoid arthritis.
58. **Acute suppurative arthritis may result due to:**
    - Blood-borne infection.
    - Local extension from some neighboring focus.
    - Direct invasion as by a penetrating injury.

59. **Recognised examples of chronic bursitis:**
    - Housemaid's knees.
    - Student's elbow.
60. **Cervical spondylolysis is characterized by:**
    - Degeneration of the intervertebral disc.
    - Formation of osteophytes.
    - Presence of neurological symptoms.
    - Formation of bony ridges running across the anterior surface of the neural canal.
61. In cases of **rheumatoid arthritis,** synovial tissue gradually encroaches upon the articular cartilage which is known as PANNUS.
62. The most common **renal complication of rheumatoid arthritis** is AMYI OIDOSIS.
63. The most disabling form of OA involves the **hip joint.**
64. **Acute polyarthritis** associated with **erythema nodosum and hilar adenopathy** occurs in SARCOIDOSIS.
65. **Olecranon bursitis** causes **student's elbow.**
66. The **ensheathing new mass of bone** in cases of **acute osteomyelitis** is known as involucrum.
67. **In cases of acute suppurative arthritis of the shoulder,** the position of ease is that of ADDUCTION.
68. The association of lymphadenopathy, splenomegaly and neutropenia with rheumatoid arthritis is known as **Felty's syndrome.**
69. **Site of maximum swelling** in cases of **acute suppurative arthritis of the elbow** is on either side of the **triceps tendon.**
70. **Bone and joint TB** is **haematogenous** in origin.
71. **Reiter's syndrome** frequently occurs in **women.**
72. CLOACAE is opening in **involucrum.**
73. The **pathological lesion of rheumatoid arthritis** is Pannus.
74. **Tuberculous abscess** of the **cervical spine** points in **supraclavicular area.**
75. Tuberculous abscess of the thoracic spine drained by→**costotransverasectomy**.
76. **Tuberculous abscess of the wrist** characteristically affects multiple joints.

Chapter ten

Metabolic Diseases of Bones and Joints

You Should Know

1. The most common cause of **osteoporosis** is →old age.
2. In **osteoporosis,** there is **a total decrease in bone volume.**
3. **Fractures** due to **senile osteoporosis** most commonly involve **vertebrae.**
4. **Osteoporosis** may result due to Cushing's syndrome, hyperthyroidism, and diabetes mellitus (DM).
5. **Postmenopausal osteoporosis** is due to lack of→OESTROGEN.
6. **Recognised feature of osteomalacia includes:**
   - Coarse thickened trabeculae on X-ray.
   - On microscopic exam in large areas of uncalcified osteoid.
   - Bilateral, symmetrical and undisplaced fracture lines.
7. **In cases of osteomalacia,** X-ray shows pseudo-fracture lines that are called LOOSER ZONES.
8. In **osteomalacia, osteoid production** is normal but mineralization is inadequate.
9. A **rachitic picture** may result due to.
   - Coeliac disease.
   - Sprue.
   - Fibrocystic disease.
10. **Renal rickets** may be caused by:
    - Chronic pyelonephritis.
    - Chronic glomerulonephritis.
    - Polycystic kidney disease.

11. **Most common cause of rickets** is inadequate intake of vitamin 'D'.
12. **Rickets may be produced by:**
    - Coeliac disease.
    - A renal defect allowing the loss of PO_4.
    - A metabolic error in alkaline phosphatase.
13. **Recognised pathology of bone in Rickets includes:**
    - Proliferation of cartilage.
    - Broad and irregular metaphysis.
    - Widening of epiphyseal line.
    - Unmolded costochondral junction.
14. **Recognised feature of Vitamin D refractory rickets includes:**
    - The child does not respond to normal dose of vitamin 'D'.
    - Large doses of vitamin 'D' are useful.
    - Most of the cases are hereditary.
15. **Increased excretion of phosphoethanolamine in urine** is a feature of **hypophosphatasia.**
16. **Recognised feature of hypophosphatasia includes:**
    - Transmitted by a recessive gene.
    - Renal calcinosis in severe forms.
    - Cranial stenosis may occur.
17. A **serum calcium** of 8 mg% and a **serum phosphorus** of **5 mg%** is found in **hypoparathyroidism.**
18. **Von Recklinghausen's disease** of **bone** is usually found in cases of a **parathyroid adenoma.**
19. **Parathormone** causes a loss of phosphatase through the kidney and an **increase in serum calcium.**
20. **"BROWN TUMOUR"** of the bone occurs in cases of **Hypoparathyroidism.**
21. **Soft tissue calcification** may be a feature of Hypophosphatasia and **Hypervitaminosis 'D'.**
22. **Recognised feature of hypothyroidism includes:**
    - Prognathous jaw.
    - Brachiocephalic skull.
    - Long bones reveal delayed bone age.
    - "Mulberry-like" epiphyseal ossification centres.

23. **In scurvy, long bones may exhibit:**
    - Subperiosteal haemorrhages.
    - Greatly reduced cartilage production.
    - Reduced osteoid formation.
    - Increased entity of the zone of provisional calcification.
    - Lateral spurrings at the ends of the shafts of the bones.
24. In **Scurvy** there is a zone of translucency on the metaphyseal side of the growth plate as seen by X-ray. This is known as zone of **fracture-dislocation.**
25. **Infantile scurvy** is generally seen only after 6 months of age.
26. **Raised serum uric acid** level is a **feature of Primary gout.**
27. **Acute inflammatory arthritis** involves one of the metatarsophalangeal joints in early stages.
28. **Recognised feature of primary gout includes:**
    - Tophi are deposited in late stages.
    - Family history are usually present.
    - Tophi are most common in the ears and about the elbows.
    - Subchondral bone destruction adjacent to the tophi.
    - Synovial fluid of the affected joint shows uric acid crystals.
29. In patients of **pseudogout, crystals of calcium pyrophosphate** are found in the **synovial fluid.**
30. **Pseudogout** results due to **deposition** of **calcium pyrophosphate crystals** within the **articular cartilage** or **soft tissue of the joint.**
31. **Ochronosis** results due to **lack of** homogentisic acid oxidase.
32. In **Ochronosis, homogentisic acid is deposited in:**
    - Sclera.
    - Tendons.
    - Joint capsule.
    - Articular cartilage.

33. The intervertebral density by X-ray in a patient of ochronosis is due to calcification of the **intervertebral disc.**
34. **Black coloured cartilage** and **tendons** are bound in→ALKAPTONURIA.
35. **Vitamin 'D' deficiency rickets** may result due to:
    - Billroth 1 gastrectomy.
    - Idiopathic sprue.
36. The **most commonly affected bone in Gaucher's disease** is→**FEMUR.**
37. **"Brown tumours"** are see in **hyperparathyroidism.**
38. The **ideal choice of a radioactive tracer** for the **study of specific cartilage** or **bone cell metabolic activity** would be an amino acid tagged with H^3, S^{35}, P^{32} or C^{12} or any of the above.
39. In **Detoni-Debre-Fanconi syndrome,** the defect is in the kidney tubular resorption of phosphates.
40. **Ochronosis** may be **misdiagnosed** with **Diabetes** due to result of urine analysis.
41. **Acromegaly is associated with:**
    - An over secretion of growth hormone.
    - Enlargement and elongation of mandible.
    - Reactivation of 'growth' at the chondro-osseous junctions.
42. **"Osteitis fibrosa"** is seen in Hyperparathyroidism and hyperthyroidism.
43. **Acceptable treatment of gout includes**— Colchicine, probenecid, phenylbutazone and salicylates in large doses.
44. **Gouty arthritis may show:**
    - Urate crystals in joint cartilage, renal glomeruli, heart valves and medullary cavity of bone.
45. **Recognised features of rickets include:**
    - Ricketary rosary.
    - Frontal bossing of skull.
    - Triradiate pelvis.
    - Bow legs.
46. **Renal rickets ensues due to:**
    - Chronic glomerulonephritis (CGN).
    - Renal tubular acidosis (RTA).

- Polycystic kidney disease (PKD).
- Chronic pyelonephritis.

47. **Wimberge line** is seen in cases of→SCRUVY.
48. The only characteristic X-ray changes of **osteomalacia** in adults is **Milkman's fractures.**
49. **Subperiosteal bone resorption** ensues in **osteitis fibrosa.**
50. **"Whiteline of Fraenkel"** is a characteristic X-ray finding of **Scurvy.**
51. The **radiological appearance of "FISH HEAD"** in the **spine** is typical of **OSTEOPOROSIS.**
52. The **classical concave "saucer" deformity** seen on radiography of the **wrist** is characteristic of **late stages of rickets.**
53. **Recognised metabolic causes of osteoporosis:**
    - Hyperthyroidism.
    - Diabetes mellitus.
    - Cushing's syndrome.
54. **Early findings of vitamin 'D' toxicity include** polyuria, polydypsia and anorexia.

Chapter eleven

Tumours of Bones and Joints

You Should Know

1. The **radioactive element** that has been observed to produce bone neoplasms in man is **Radon (Ra^{286}).**
2. **Bone tumours arising from cartilage include:**
   - Osteochondroma.
   - Osteoblstoma.
   - Chondromyxoid fibroma.
   - Enchondroma.

Note: Chondroblastoma is not a tumour arising from cartilage.

3. **Enchondroma** is a **true tumour.**
4. The commonest bony lesion in children below the age of five year is **neuroblastoma.**
5. **Fibrosarcoma of bone** is classified as **true neoplasm.**
6. **Regarding osteoid osteoma:**
   - Nidus surrounded by an area of reactive bone are characteristic radiographic features.
   - Nidus is highly vascular.
   - Surgical excision of the lesion is the treatment of choice.
7. The **size of osteoid osteoma** is not more than **1 cm.**
8. A **benign tumour** forming osteoid is an **osteoma.**
9. **Osteoid osteoma** is mostly found in the age group of **10 to 25 years.**
10. **The osteoid osteoma may originate in:**
    - The bone cortex.
    - The periosteum.

- The medullary cavity.
- The junction of endosteum and the bone cortex.

11. Commonest site of **Ivory osteoma** is **skull bone**.
12. Vertebrae is mostly involved by **osteoblastoma**.
13. **Osteoblastoma** does not show characteristic X-ray pattern.
14. An **osteoblastoma** is easily most confused by X-ray and histologically with **osteosarcoma**.
15. **Histologic feature of osteosarcomas includes:**
    - The lesion consists of highly vascular osteoid.
    - There is abundane of osteoblasts.
    - Areas of actual bone formation are evident.
16. **Regarding osteoclastoma:**
    - Is very rarely malignant.
    - Is common in females than in males.
    - Characteristically occurs in the shaft of a long bone.
    - Subperiosteal new bone is demonstrable radiologically.
17. A enzyme present in the osteoclast but absent in the osteoblast is→**ACID PHOSPHATASE**.
18. **"Soap bubble"** or **"Mosaic appearance"** on radiological examination is characteristic of→Osteoclastoma.
19. **Osteoclastoma** may resemble **osteitis fibrocystica.**
20. **Regarding osteogenic sarcoma:**
    - Usually metastasizes by the bloodstream.
    - Has an age range of less than five years to over fifty.
    - Is a tumour in which true multicentric lesions may simultaneously arise.
    - Has a highly characteristic X-ray picture.
21. **The most common primary osseous malignant tumour** is→OSTEOGENIC SARCOMA.
22. The **commonest site of osteosarcoma** is **upper end of FEMUR.**
23. **Regarding osteogenic sarcoma:**
    - Are frequently surrounded by non-malignant new bone formation.
    - Readily metastasises via the bloodstream.

- Are most frequent in the 10 to 25 years age group.

24. **Radiologic feature of osteogenic sarcoma may include:**
    - Scattered island of bone.
    - Codman's triangle.
    - Pathologic fracture.
    - Sun-ray appearance.
25. The **most common type of osteosarcoma** is radiating spicule type.
26. The **initial treatment of osteogenic sarcoma** is radical amputation.
27. **Osteosarcoma** carrying poorest prognosis is **sarcoma of Paget's disease.**
28. The commonest site of metastases in cases of osteosarcoma is **lung.**
29. ENCHONDROMA is best treated by **subperiosteal resection.**
30. The **commonest site of enchondroma** is long tubular bones of the hands and feet.
31. **Regarding enchondroma.**
    - The tumour is often calcified.
    - It is a cartilagenous tumour.
    - Pathological fracture may result.
32. **Regarding multiple hereditary osteochondroma:**
    - More common in males.
    - Transmitted as a dominant trait.
    - Growth disturbances are present.
    - There is generalized involvement throughout the body.
33. X-ray picture of **chondromyxoid fibroma** most closely **resembles** non-osteogenic fibroma.
34. **Recognised components of chondromyxoid fibroma include:**
    - Chondroid.
    - Myxoid.
    - Fibroid.
35. **Chondromyxoid fibroma** most commonly seen in the metaphysis of the long bones.

36. A condition of multiple enchondromatosis along with multiple hemangiomas in **Maffucci's syndrome.**
37. **Chondroblastomas** occur mostly in the age group **10 to 20 years.**
38. The most characteristic histologic feature of **chondroblastoma is→calcification.**
39. **Chondroblastoma** typically involves the **epiphyses of the long bones.**
40. **Radiotherapy** is of **least value** in **chondrosarcoma.**
41. A lesion known to extend directly into regional blood vessels and expand on plugs in the vessel lumen without adhesion to the vessel walls is **chondrosarcoma.**
42. The incidence of **chondrosarcoma** developing in a patient having **multiple osteochondromatosis** is **15%.**
43. **Recognised feature of chondrosarcoma includes:**
    - Painful bony swelling.
    - Swelling is tender.
    - Metastases may occur into lungs.
    - Spread through blood vessels is common.
44. **Recognised feature of fibrous cortical defect includes:**
    - Foam cells and multinucleate giant cells are often presents within the lesion.
    - Usually asymptomatic.
    - Surgery is not indicated.
45. **Regarding non-ossifying fibroma** on X-ray it gives pseudoloculated radiolucent defect in the bone.
46. The combination of blotchy, skin pigmentation, fibrous dysplasia and premature sexual development in the female is termed as **Albright's syndrome.**
47. Regarding **fibrosarcomata of the bone,** it will demonstrate bone destruction with no new bone formation on X-ray.

48. **Characteristic X-ray of a fibrosarcoma of bone includes:**
    - Similar to those of giant cell tumour.
    - Similar to those of Ewing's sarcoma.
    - Similar to those of an inflammatory lesion.
    - Primarily a lytic lesion destroying bone.
49. **Aneurysmal bone cysts are almost certainly non-neoplastic.**
50. Among fibrosarcoma, osteosarcoma and chondrosarcoma, **fibrosarcoma is** the **least common.**
51. **Regarding unicamral bone cyst:**
    - Usually seen in metaphyses of long bone.
    - Contains a straw coloured fluid.
    - One of the commonest bony lesion.
    - Psedoloculation are frequently present.
52. Most common site for a **solitary bone cyst** is **metaphyses.**
53. **Regarding Adamantinoma of bone radiologically:**
    - May be confused with cortical fibrous dysplasias.
    - May involve one or more bone.
    - Appears as a lytic lesion involving a cortex of bone.
    - Characteristically has a polycystic appearance.
54. **Adamantinoma** is **most common** in the **MANDIBLE.**
55. **Microscopically histiocytosis shows:**
    - Multiple eosinophils.
    - Masses of histiocytes filled with cholesterol.
    - Scarring and sclerosis in old lesions.
56. **Osseous hemangiomas** are most common in the **vertebral bodies.**
57. **Regarding giant cell tumour of bone (osteoclastoma):**
    - Occurs in epiphysis of the long bones.
    - There is a malignant potential.
    - Surgical excision, if possible, is the treatment of choice.
58. Microscopic feature of **giant cell tumour** is indistinguishable from those of Brown tumour of hyperparathyroidism.

59. Treatment of choice for giant cell tumour is **total excision.**
60. **Reed-Sternberg giant cells** are diagnostic of **Hodgkin's disease.**
61. Radiographic punched out lesions of bone with minimal reactive sclerosis are characteristic of **multiple myeloma.**
62. **BJP** (Bence-Jons-Protein) in the urine is found in cases of→**Multiple myeloma.**
63. **Paget's disease** is also called **osteitis deformans.**
64. **Regarding Paget's disease of bone:**
    - Femur, tibia and spine are involved commonly.
    - There is skull bone thickening and deformity.
    - Serum alkaline phosphatase is raised.
    - Osteogenic sarcoma is common.
65. **Paget's disease** is most likely to degenerate into an →**Osteosarcoma.**
66. **Regarding Ewing's sarcoma of bone:**
    - Occurs in metaphysis of long bone.
    - Occurs in early age groups.
    - X-ray shows "onion-peel" appearance due to layers of new subperiosteal bone formation.
    - Has poor prognosis.
67. **Differential diagnosis of Ewing's tumour includes:**
    - Metastatic granuloma.
    - Reticulum cell sarcoma.
    - Chronic osteomyelitis.
68. **Regarding tumours resembling primary reticulum cell sarcoma of bone** clinically or histologically includes:
    - Ewing's sarcoma.
    - Neuroblastoma.
    - Leukaemia.
    - Lymphoma.
69. **Reticulum cell sarcoma of bone** usually affects only one bone.
70. **Rosettes** are formed in NEUROBLASTOMA.
71. A metastatic tumour best known for its **osteoblastic bone reaction** is from **C_A prostate gland.**

72. The most common metastatic tumour to bone is from C_A **breast.**
73. **"Onion-peel" appearance** is characteristic of **Ewing's tumour.**
74. **Leukaemia** affects osseous areas most frequently at epiphyseal-metaphyseal junction.
75. **An osteoid osteoma:**
    - Commonly presents with local pain.
    - Demonstrates a small circular band of long sclerosis surrounding a translucent area on X-ray.
76. **Metastatic lesions of bone:**
    - Often simulate primary bone tumours.
    - Are rare distal to knee or elbow.
77. **Malignant degeneration** of **benign bone lesion** following X-ray therapy has been observed in:
    - Giant cell tumour.
    - Solitary bone cyst.
    - Normal bone.
    - Fibrous dysplasia.
    - Chondroblastoma.
78. **Regarding benign tumors of cartilage:**
    - Chondromata and osteochondromata occur equally in both sexes.
    - Malignant changes occur in 10% of cases of multiple osteochondromata.
79. **Regarding chodrosarcoma:**
    - Is about 50% as common as osteosarcoma.
    - May be histologically malignant in the hand or foot yet be clinically benign.
    - Is usually the correct diagnosis in an adult with a growing cartilagenous lesion.
80. **Clinically Ewing's tumour may present:**
    - A temperature curve of a septic type.
    - A common finding of referred pain.
    - Local pain and a palpable mass.
    - Anaemia and leukocytosis.
    - Symptom of upto one year duration.
81. **Recognised features associated with non-ossifying fibromas of bone:**
    - Microscopically they characteristically contain foam cells.

- They appear at onset 1.5 to 2 cm. away from the growth plate.
- Are eccentrically positioned in the bone.

82. **Regarding Desmoplastic fibromas of bone:**
    - Is closely associated with/in histology with fibrosarcoma.
    - Require vigorous surgical excision and justifies segmental resection.
83. **Regarding chondrosarcoma:**
    - Commonly invade the neighbouring blood vessels.
    - Those which develop in the metaphysis are usually less well differentiated than those occurring around the epiphysis.
84. **Regarding giant cell tumour (osteoclastoma):**
    - May metastasize while appearing benign by microscope.
    - May be closely simulated in hyperparathyroidism.
85. **Predisposing factors for osteogenic sarcoma** include:
    - Excessive irradiation.
    - Paget's disease.
86. **Bone tumours presents** as:
    - A cause of pain.
    - A noticeable lump.
    - A pathologic fracture.
    - A tender area.
87. Osteoclastoma of a rib should be treated by excision of part or whole bone.
88. **Codman's triangle** is due to subperiosteal new bone deposition seen in osteosarcoma.
89. **Osteoid osteoma** is most common in **femur** and **tibia.**
90. **Chondrosarcoma** has a predilection for the small bone and ribs.
91. The **giant cell tumour** gives a typical **soap bubble appearance** on radiography.
92. **Chondroma** is most frequent in metacarpals, phalanges and metatarsals.
93. **Ivory osteoma** arises from the membrane bone of the **skull.**

94. **Paget's disease** predispose bone to develop **sarcoma.**
95. **Second most common malignant tumour** of **bone** is **chondrosarcoma.**
96. In **Enchondroma,** there is thin and expanded cortex.
97. **Most common malignant tumour of bone** is **multiple myeloma**.

Chapter twelve

Recent Advances in Ortho-Diagnostic Radiology

INTRODUCTION

The **modernisation of diagnostic radiology** is based on **X-ray technology.** It utilises the contrast media like air, gas or I_2 based solutions. With the help of such contrast media, we are able to delineate the cavities, tract, sinuses, spaces and know their dimensions, extent, etc.

> ***Note:*** *The air and gases are less irritant, less toxic, miscible, and easily absorbed or excreted. While the iodine containing compounds are irritants, toxic, non-miscible and slowly absorbable. Metrizamide is the most commonly used contrast media.*

I. INVASIVE DIAGNOSIS

The following types of investigation uses contrast media in orthopedics.

a. Arthrography is the process of visualising the interior of the joint by injecting contrast liquid into the joint.

   Indications:

   - To know the damage of intra-articular structure, as for example ACL, meniscal tears in knee.
   - To confirm the loosening of the prosthesis where the dye will percolate around the loosened-loosened stem, i.e. bone cement interface.
   - To confirm the capsular tear, etc.

- To utline the intra-articular cartilaginous structure, e.g. femoral head in CDH.
- **Arthrography** which is done by injecting iodinated contrast and air into the joint, followed by conventional radiographs in different projection.

  Arthrography is the radiologic examination of joint to demonstrate its internal anatomy using single or double contrast media.

> *Note: Although any synovial joint can be evaluated by this method it is usually done for large joints like hip, knee and shoulder joints.*

- Conray 280/urogafin 60% approximately 4 to 10 ml in amount depending on the joint to be evaluated.
- Air is used for double contrast study, sometimes only air may be used to delineate the synovial cavity. Such type of procedure is called **pneumo-arthrography.**

Preliminary Films

a. Shoulder joint—AP, lateral and additional views like axial views, Stryker's views may be required for evaluation of recurrent dislocation.
b. Knee joint—AP and lateral views.
c. Hip joint—AP and lateral views. Additional view like von Rosen's view may be required for evaluation of CDH in children.

Technique

Under LA, a needle through all aseptic technique inserted into the joint space. In cases of synovial effusion, fluid is aspirated and the contrast medium followed by air is injected. The joint is gently exercised to allow even distribution of the contrast.

Film taken like preliminary films for knee joint, besides stress films are taken under fluoroscopic control to evaluated for meniscal/ligamentous injuries. Films taken half an hour later may be invaluable for demonstration of intra-articular loose bodies as contrast gets absorbed on their surface, permitting/allowing better demonstration.

- Before NMR/MRI, arthrography was done routinely for evaluation of suspected meniscal or cruciate ligament tears and for diagnosis of rotator cuff tears.
- MRI is noninvasive offers superior anatomic information and diagnoses these injuries with greater accuracy than arthrography.

> ***Note:*** *Currently, arthrography is rarely done, it is kept reserved for those patients in which MRI/NMR is contraindicated.*

b. *Discography* is the process whereby contrast material is injected into the intervertebral disc. It is usually indicated to diagnose the disc degeneration and prolapse disc.

c. *Sinography* is a process whereby a contrast material is introduced inside the sinus tract through its ostia. It is used to know the directin, extent, source and possible cause of such sinuses.

d. *Facetography* is the process in which contrast dye is injected into the facet joints. It is used to delineate the abnormalities of the facet joints and rupture of the facet joint capsule.

e. *Myelography and radioculography:* These days these procedures are usually combined with CT. Post-myelogram CT or myelo. CT or even MRI scan. Here contrast liquid is introduced into the sub-arachnoid space.
   - It is used to delineate any pressure on the spinal cord and roots, e.g. extramedullary spinal cord and roots.
   - Intervertebral disc herniation.
   - To know the dimension of the vertebral canal, e.g. vertebral canal stenosis.

f. *Discogram:* Under fluoroscopic or CT guidance, a contrast media is injected into a suspected symptomatic disc to attempt to reproduce the patient's symptoms exactly. This provocative test is particularly useful for patients who have several potentially symptomatic abnormal discs or a single abnormal disc or doubtful significane.

> ***Note:*** *A discogram is rarely indicated and its use is controversial. Besides, the results of the test are somewhat subjective and can be difficult to interpret. It is, infact, of limited specificity. The above procedure from "a to f" are also called INVASIVE.*

II. NON-INVASIVE DIAGNOSIS

- These also include various methodology like ultrasonography, tomography, xeroradiography, CAT scan, MRI scan, scientigraphy etc.

  Ultrasound or USG (Ultrasonography) can be used for diagnostic as well as therapeutic purposes.

  Principle: The ultrasonography is based on the principle of recording of reflection of soundwaves from the resistnaces of different densities. The reflected sound is converted into an image. It utilises piezoelectric crystals to produce such high frequency sound waves. The tissues of different densities can be reproduced as images in gradation of grey, which can reasonably delineate the anatomical outline.
- According human tissues are classified into echogenicity as:
  - Highly echogenic—mostly solid, e.g. Fat.
  - Mildly echogenic—semisolid tissues.
  - Echo free—fluid filled cystic structure.

Uses of USG

i. Due to contrast echogenicity of solid vs cystic masses, USG is mainly useful in diagnosing the deep seated cystic lesions like cysts, abscesses, haematoma, aneurysm, intra-articular fluids, etc.

ii. USG is almost routinely used to screen the newborn for CDH (congenital dislocation of hip).

> ***Note:*** *USG may well demarcate the relation between acetabular labrum and cartilaginous femoral head epiphysis.*

iii. USG may be helpful in diagnosing the rotator cuff injuries of the shoulder joint, and internal derangements of the knee.

> ***Note:*** *However, the interpretation may be difficult and even inaccurate.*

Tomography

It is the X-ray image focussed on a desired plane. By rotating the tube and the X-ray film in opposite direction on any imaginary pivot, the pictures produced on either side of the pivotal plane are blurred out. Pictures obtained on different plane cuts, reveal the lesions which are obscured on plane X-rays.

Uses

a. It can be useful in classifying the vague and obscured findings of plane X-rays of occult injuries. It can assist in further assessment of a known *fracture* or *fracture dislocation.*
b. In *spinal region,* it is very useful for identifying the facet fractures and the obscured defects in the parts interarticularis.
c. It also reveals the deep seated lesions like osteoid osteoma, brodies abscess, infective focus, etc.
d. It may help identify a less obvious sequestrum or subchondral bony plate destruction in septic arthritis and thus distinguish it from periarticular osteoporosis, where the subchondral plate remains intact.

III. XERORADIOGRAPHY

Xeroradiography also utilizes the X-ray exposure as done to evaluate anything routinely. Here, the response is registered as an electrically changed pattern on the recording plate, which is reproduced in the form of positive images on a plastic coated paper. The photoelectrical process involved here is mainly sensitive to variations in the tissue density.

- Recognised uses of xeroradiography includes vague, obscured and fuzzy lesions, e.g.
- Subperiosteal erosions (early osteomyelitis)

- Early soft tissue calcification (myositis ossification)
- Early cartilaginous calcification (chondrocalcinosis) etc. may displayed not only more easily but also earlier than by the use of the plane X-rays.

IV. CAT SCAN

> ***Note: Douglas Hounsfeld (1974)*** *discovered CAT scan machine.*

- CAT scan produces transaxial cutting images through selected tissue planes, by which the anatomical planes, not delineable by plane X-rays, can be easily demonstrated.
- Firstly a 'survey view' of the region is taken in which the affected area is selected and through it a series of cross-sectional iamges are obtained cutting slices are usually 5 to 10 mm apart, when done through the bigger joints or the tissues.

> ***Note:*** *However, much thinner slices are cut in cases of small joints, intervertebral disc or smaller tissues, etc.*

- With the help of special equipment, different transaxial cut images are made in coronal or sagittal or even 3D images of bones having complicated shapes like vertebrae, thus enhances its utility in delineating such structure.
- **CAT scan** has proved to be a very useful diagnostic aid in evaluating anatomical dimensions of spinal canal, spinal trauma and diseases of the areas.
- **Canal stenosis**—The standard CT scan suggest foraminal narrowing. It is also useful in defining the lateral recess stenosis and foraminal stenosis, which is hardly possible in myelography.
- **CT is helpful in** assessing the degree of encroachment of spinal canal by a fractured fragment, herniated intervertebral disc or any other space occupying lesion. The best way of confirming the diagnosis is by metrizamide or iohexol myelography combined with a reformatted CAT scan of the

suspected segment. Combined with MRI/NMR, post-myelogram contrast CT can suggest 96 to 97% **accurate diagnosis**.

> *Note:* ***Radiation exposure*** *involves* ***4.8 to 7 rads*** *and the need for an invasive procedure for injecting the dye are disadvantages of contrast CT.*

- **Spinal trauma:** Fractures of cervicothoracic and thoracic or thoracolumbar regions may be missed on plane X-rays. Injuries to osseous, ligamentous and neurological structures can be evaluated with a high degree of accuracy through the sophisticated imaging technique like tomography, contrast myelography, postmyelogram CT with sagittal reconstruction and MRI scan.
- **CAT** is helpful in assessing the degree of compromise of the spinal canal. Reformatted CT scans of the cervical spine usually present less distinct picture than in the lumbar spine.
- **Spinal infections:** The findings of **CAT scan** is more or less similar to those of plane X-rays including the lytic lesions in the subchondral zone, destruction of the end plate, sclerosed margin of the lytic lesions, lesser density and flattening of the disc, disruptin of bone in the paradiscal and peridiscal region, soft tissues shadows in epidural, paravertebral and paraspinal areas and abscesses.

> *Note:* ***Postmyelogram CAT scan*** *clearly difines the compression of the spinal cord and other neural elements by abscess or sequestrum or bone or other materials.*

- **Spinal tumours—CAT scan** is of much use in **assessing** the **size, shape and infiltration** of the **neoplasms. Postmyelo-CT clearly defines the SOL in vertebral canal.**
- CT can't demonstrate intraspinal tumours (unlike MRI) and arachnoiditis. It also can't differentiate between old scars and new disc herniation.
- CT is a very sensitive investigation for detecting pulmonary metastases in malignant tumours.

> *Note:* ***Myelography*** *along with* ***multiplanner CAT scan scars*** *may be of much use in evaluating the intraspinal and extraspinal effects of spondylolisthesis including disc herniation.*

- **Fractures not clearly defined in plane X-ray can be well displayed by CAT scan.**
- **High resolution CAT scan** is very useful in meniscal tears.

> *Note:* ***CAT scan*** *can be used in assessing the patellofemoral joint, synovial cysts and soft tissue tumours in and around the knee joint.*

V. MAGNETIC RESONANCE IMAGING (MRI)

- **Felix Bloch** and **EM Purcell (1946)** discovered the physical phenomenon of **MRI**, based upon assessment of radiofrequency emissions from atoms and molecules in tissues, exposed to an external magnetic field.

> *Note:* ***Odebald and Lindstrom (1955)*** *pioneered the medical application of NMR.*

- **Damadian and Hinslow (1977)** were the 1st to produce the NMR images.
- The images recorded in MRI are more or less similar to those of CT scans, but have more clarity and tissue contrast. The sectional images can be produced in any plane, and reconstituted to project **3D pictures.**
- The intensity of MRI signal depends upon the concentration of H_2 nuclei in the tissues underscanning and their spinning character and relaxation rates following protein excitation.
- The physical phenomenon of relaxation is expressed by two independent tissue constants T_1 and T_2, producing two signal simultaneously.
- The **T_1-weighted** images are sharp, well defined and almost anatomical in appearance.

- The **T_2-weighted** images project more of the pathological character of the tissues.
- Tissue with maximum concentration of **H_2 nuclei** unit high intensity signals producing the brightest images (e.g. fat, bone-marrow, cancellous bone, etc), those with little concentration of H_2 unit low intensity signal projected as black (e.g. ligaments, bony cortex, tendons, air, etc) and those with intermediate concentration are produced in the grey scale (e.g. cartilage muscle, spinal canal, etc).

> ***Note:*** *Other frequently used pulse sequences are proton density and shorter invasion recovery (STIR), which has the property to suppress the signals from fat and increase the contrast for* ***H_2O*** *containing tissues.*

- **Recognised use of MRI (NMR)**
- **MRI is marginally superior to spine myelo-CT in identifying the spinal lesion.** It can suitably examine the entire spine, identifying the degenerated disc, delineate the cord and root impingement, demonstrate the intra-spinal tumours and evaluate the thecal space and tissues in the foramen.
- **Spinal infections** can be identified quickly and more or less accurately.

> ***Note:*** *MRI can't differentiate between the pyogenic and non-pyogenic infection.*

- The calcifications in tuberculous abscess are not identified in MRI. While it is well demonstrated in plain X-ray.
- **Spinal injuries.**
  - MRI has a definite role in early detection of the avascular necrosis of femoral head.
  - **In carpal tunnel syndrome,** the synovial disease, narrowing of the tunnel and median nerve compression can be well delineate in MRI.
- **MRI is likely to be a very accurate** investigation for assessing the extent of bone and soft tissue involvement by the tumour.

Recognised advantages of MRI include

a. It is non-invasive, versatile, and sensitive technique with fairly high degree of specificity and accuracy and with no risk of ionizing radiation.
b. It does not require frequent repositioning as in myelography.
c. It produces clear and high soft tissue contrast differentiating the bone and soft tissues.

Disadvantages of MRI include

a. Not a cost-effective investigation (very-very expensive).
b. Require the patient to lie still in a particular position, which can become painful and annoying.
c. The fear of remaining in a closed vessel for a long period (claustrophobia) may create a problem and hence affecting the final result of MRI.
d. It is contraindicated in persons having **pacemakers implant** replaced **joints** or **implants.**

VI. SCINTIGRAPHY (RADIOACTIVE ISOTOPE OR RADIONUCLIDES STUDIES)

Introduction

Different tissues take up radioisotopes according to their activities and emit photons which can be recorded by simple rectilinear scanner or a gamma camera to produce an image.

> ***Note:*** *In orthopaedics, radionucleides commonly used are Tc-99m, Gallium 67, Technetium labelled sulphur colloid Indium-111-labelled leucocytes.*

- Technetium-99m has been found to be the ideal for radionuclide imaging.
- Recently-99m-Tc-HDP (Technitium labelled hydroxymethelene diphosphonate) is used IV and uptake activities are recorded in 3 phases.
  a. The "flow phase": It is akin to radionuclide angiogram demonstrating the blood flow.

b. Immediate or perfusion or equilibrium or "blood pool" phase: Immediately after the injection, the image shows relative vascular flow and distribution of radioisotope in the perivascular and extracellular space.
c. *Delayed or bone phase:* Two to 4 hours after the injection, when most of the isotope has been excreted, except that taken up in the bone by its osteoblastic activities.

- Normally in the **equilibrium phase,** the periarticular vascular tissues take up the isotope most actively and produce darkest images, which gradually fade away. **Two to 4 hours later** in the **"delayed phase"** the uptake is more in the metaphyseal cancellous area showing more activity, and the outlines of bone are shown more clearly.
- **Abnormal recordings** of the uptake are significant when it is sharply localised or obviously assymetrical. Broadly the abnormal recordings can be of 4 types:
  a. **Incresed uptake** in the equilibrium or perfusion phase. It indicates increased vascularity of the soft tissues, e.g. in acute (or even chronic) inflammatory changes.
  b. **Decreased uptake** in 'equilibrium phase'. It indicates decreased vascularity of the soft tissues. It is an unusual finding.
  c. **Increased uptake in delayed phase:** It indicates increased activities in the ECG or more precisely in the process of new bone formation in fracture healing, inflammation of bone, bone tumours, revascularisation in osteonecrosis, myositic activities and heterotropic bone formation.
- **Osteomyelitis focus** usually presents as an area of increased tracer uptake **(hot area)**, but in infants, due to oedematous occlusion of the intramedullary vessels, these decreased delivery of the isotope leading to decreased tracer uptake **(cold spot or area).**
- The **tracer (^{99m}Tc)** uptake will be more in the active bone tumours, bone involvements in malignant soft tissue tumours and occult bone metastases.

d. Decreased uptake in **"delayed" phase**. It indicates decreased vascularity of the bone, e.g. in avascular necrosis of femoral head, fibrotic replacement of bony tissues, etc.

- **Recognised uses of Scintigraphy**
    - Early detection of **acute osteomyelitis** focus and bony abscess.
    - Early detection of bony metastasis.
    - Detection and localisation of **avascular necrosis of bone.** (e.g. Perthes disease, idiopathic osteonecrosis, avascular necrosis following fractures, etc).
    - Early detection of **stress fracture.**
    - Detection of **degenerative joint diseases.**
    - Detection of infection in **prosthetic implant.**

Immunoscintigraphy

- Here in this technique, the radioactive labelled antibodies, directed against tumour associated surface antigens, are injected IV and the site of the ag-ab reaction is located and imaged by recording the emitted **X-rays** with the help of γ (gamma) camera.

> *Note: The development of **monoclonal antibodies** and the possibilities of labelling them with **short-lived technetium** has significantly increased the use of immunoscintigraphy in clinical practice.*

- Currently immunoscintigraphy is being utilized for making **specific diagnosis of recurrent** and **metastasis** in **colorectal C_A** and other **tumours producing CEA, ovarian C_A, lymphomas and melanomas, etc.**

Chapter thirteen

Most Common in Orthopaedics Worth Remembering

You Should Know

1. **Dislocation of spine** is most common at → C5 and C6
2. Most commonly **"Herring bone pattern"** is seen in → Fibrosarcoma
3. Most commonly **"Bucket handle tear"** ensues in injury due to → Menisci of knee joint
4. Most common complication of **shoulder dislocation is** → Injury to **Axillary Nerve**
5. Most common bony lesion of hyperparathyroidism is found in → Jaws
6. Most common cause of **non-union in fracture is** → Lack of adequate immobilization
7. Treatment of choice for **acute myositis ossificans is** → Immobilization
8. **Avascular necrosis of femoral head** is most commonly seen in: → Subcapital fracture
9. **Tenosynovitis of ring finger** most commonly spread to → Midpalmar space
10. **Slipped femoral epiphysis** is most commonly seen in the → 2nd decade
11. Most common site of **multiple myeloma is** → Vertebra
12. Most commonly **nerve abscess in leprosy** are seen in the → Ulnar nerve
13. **Myositis ossificans** is most commonly seen at the → Elbow joint
14. Most common organism causing osteomyelitis in children under 3 years of age is → *H. influenzae*
15. Most common site of **acute osteomyelitis in infant** is → Upper end of femur

16.	**Herbeden nodes** at distal interphalangeal joints are seen most commonly in	→ Osteoarthritis
17.	**Dislocation of knee joint** is most commonly due to	→ Rupture of cruciate ligament
18.	**"Sun ray appearance"** on X-ray most commonly seen in	→ Osteogenic sarcoma
19.	Most common **pain sensitive structure** in a **joint** is	→ Fibrous capsule
20.	**Meyer's operation** is most commonly done for	→ Fracture neck femur
21.	Pyogenic osteomyelitis of the spine is mostly caused by	→ Pseudomonas
22.	Earliest C/M of spinal TB is	→ **Muscle spasm**
23.	Pain in Paget's disease is best relieved by	→ **Calcitonin**
24.	Most common **"fish mouth appearance"** of the vertebral bodies is seen in	→ Osteoporosis
25.	Tissue most sensitive to radiation is	→ Epiphysis.
26.	**Chemical synovectomy** is mostly done by	→ Osmic acid
27.	Most commonly **fat embolism** is associated with	→ Petechial haemorrhages
28.	**Bleeding into joint cavities** is least (not) common in	→ ITP
29.	Most common age group for **osteogenic sarcoma** is	→ 10 to 20 years
30.	Most common **epiphyseal tumour** in children is	→ Chondroblastoma
31.	The earliest feature of **Pott's paraplegia** is	→ **Ankle clonus**
32.	Most commonly **foot drop** results from	→ **Common peroneal nerve palsy**
33.	A ruptured nerve with untidy wound is best sutured in	→ **Two to three weeks**
34.	Most commonly **compound fracture** is a fracture with involvement of	→ Skin or cutis
35.	Mostly nerve suturing in a clear cut injury is done in	→ Six hours
36.	Radiation is least likely to cause	→ Fibrosarcoma

37. Most commonly a radio-opaque line is seen at the metaphysis in	→	**Lead poisoning**
38. Most commonly in **gout,** crystal consists of	→	**MSU** (monosodium urate)
39. Most commonly **Pott's fracture is a**	→	**Bimalleolar fracture**
40. Most common cause of internal disturbance of knee joint is	→	**Medial meniscal injury**
41. In **bone grafting,** bone is mostly taken from	→	Ileum
42. **Myositis ossificans** is most commonly seen in fracture of	→	Supracondylar humerus
43. Most commonly bone growth is influenced maximally by	→	Testosterone
44. Most commonly in **trochanteric fracture** early mobilization can be achieved using	→	Blade, plate, and screws
45. Most commonly **axillary nerve injury** at its origin led to paralysis of	→	Deltoid and teres minor
46. **Injury to the popliteal artery** in fracture lower end of femur is most often due to	→	Distal fragment pressing the artery
47. Most commonly **"sabre tibia"** is seen in	→	Congenital syphilis
48. Most common site of **ivory osteoma** is	→	Frontal sinus
49. Most commonly **fibrous dysplasia of bone** with precocious puberty and pigmentation is seen in	→	Albright syndrome
50. Most commonly **complete claw hand** results due to injury to	→	Ulnar and median nerve
51. The nerve most commonly involved in **Tarsal tunnel syndrome** is	→	Posterior tibial
52. Most commonly **Bouchard's nodes** are seen at the	→	Proximal interphalangeal joint

53. Most common cause of **scoliosis** besides idiopathic, in children is → Post polio myelitis
54. Most commonly peripheral nerves resist ischaemia upto → 1 hour
55. Most common cause of **neuropathic joints** is → Diabetes mellitus
56. The most common site of **aneurysmal bone cyst is** → Upper end of tibia
57. **"Nail patella syndrome"** is mostly characterized by → Nephritis
58. Most commonly fraying at the ends of long bones is seen in → **Rickets**
59. In adults, Achilles tendon most commonly ruptures spontaneously at → 3 cm above attachment with calcaneus
60. **Osseous metastasis** is most common if tumour is in → BRONCHUS
61. Most common cause of **anterior compartment** syndrome is → **Postischemic swelling**
62. **Intraosseous skeletal tumour** is best diagnosed by → **MRI or NMR**
63. **Organism most commonly** found in **chronic osteomyelitis** is → *Staph. aureus*
64. **Metaphyseal fracture** is most commonly seen in → **Scurvy**
65. **Normal disc space** with collapseof $L_{2,3}$ is most commonly seen in → **Malignancy**
66. **Fall on hell with fracture OS calcis** is associated most commonly with → **Fracture vertebra**
67. **Vertebral disc prolapse** with intact vertebra pedicles seen most commonly in → **Trauma**
68. **Frost bite arthritis** resembles most commonly to → **Rheumatoid arthritis**
69. Best skin cover in complete avulsion of heel is → **Myocutaneous flap**
70. Most commonly **"Patellar tap"** is diagnostic of → **Knee effusion**

71. The most common **elbow injury** in children is	→ Extension type of supracondylar fracture of humerus
72. Mostly **Volkmann's ischaemic** contracture is due to:	→ Increase of compartment pressure in the limb
73. Most commonly **Klumpke's paralysis is** due to injury of:	→ Medial cord of brachial plexus
74. **Turn-graft operation** is most commonly done in femur.	→ Osteoclastoma of lower end
75. Most commonly **Morrant Baker cyst** is seen in	→ Monoarticular rheumatoid arthritis
76. Most commonly **"brown tumours"** are seen in	→ Hyperparathyroidism
77. Most commonly **"Tinel's sign"** is seen in	→ **Nerve regeneration**
78. The **most common site of chondroma in vertebral column** is	→ Thoracic region
79. The term **"orthropaedics"** was coined by	→ **Nicholas Andrey**
80. Most commonly night cries are seen in children with	→ **T.B. arthritis**
81. Most common complication of **Colles' fracture is**	→ **Malunion**
82. Most common site for **Meningocele** is	→ **Lumbosacral**
83. Bone metastasis is best diagnosed by	→ **Radioisotope scan**
84. Most commonly Tennis elbow presents as	→ **Pain over lateral epicondyle**
85. **Flattening of pedicles of vertebra** occurs most commonly in	→ Intraspinal tumour
86. In **posterolateral disc prolapse,** the disc ruptures mostly through	→ **Annulus fibrosus**
87. Most commonly **neuropathic joint** is seen in	→ **Syphilitic arthritis**
88. Earliest sign of infection in **multiple pinning** done for fracture neck femur is	→ Rarefaction around pin

89. Most commonly **"Pop corn" calcification** is seen in → **Chondrosarcoma**
90. Most commonly **"Egawa test"** is done for → **Dorsal interossei**
91. **"Bone in bone appearance"** is seen most commonly in → **Rickets or osteopetrosis**
92. Most commonly juxta articular demineralization is seen in → **Rheumatoid arthritis**
93. **Widening of metaphysis of meta-carpal** is seen most commonly in → Acromegaly
94. Most commonly **Klippel Fiel syndrome** is due to → Segmentation defect of cervical spine
95. **Hematogenous osteomyelitis** is most commonly seen around → **Knee joint**
96. **Dislocation of head of radius** (pulled elbow) is most common in children because of → **Rupture of Annular cartilage**
97. The most common tumour that cause intradural extramedullary block in spinal canal is → **Neurofibroma**
98. **Most important pathology in club foot** is → Congenital talonavicular dislocation
99. Most common site of **fracture in senile osteoporosis** is → Vertebra
100. Most **common type of shoulder dislocation is** → **Subcoracoid**
101. **Multiple short long bones of hand and foot** are most commonly infected by → **Tuberculosis**
102. **Epiphyseal injuries** are most common in the region of → **Wrist**
103. When the spine is involved in metastatic disease, the most frequent site of primary is → **Breast**
104. Type of **osteosarcoma** that carries **poorest prognosis** is → Paget's disease
105. The aetiology of **rheumatoid arthritis** is best explained at present as a disorder of → **Immune mechanism**
106. The bone most frequently involved by **actinomycosis osteomyelitis** is → **Mandible**

107. **Angioma of muscles** is mostly found in → **Rectus femoris**
108. If several ribs are fractured both anteriorly and posteriorly early death is most often due to → **Flail chest**
109. The most common site of epiphyseal plate injuries is reported to be at the → **Wrist**
110. The most common early complication of major hip surgery is → **Haematoma**
111. Treatment of the early clubfoot is best performed by → **Plaster casts**
112. In the **Nail-Patella syndrome** the most common associated deformity is → **Shape of pelvis**
113. Most important predisposing lesion to **primary bone tumour** is → **Knee joint**
114. The joint least likely to have **recurrent dislocation** is → **Knee joint**
115. The earliest destructive anatomical changes in rheumatoid arthritis begin in the → **Attachment of the capsule**
116. Most common cause of **Pes cavus** is → **Poliomyelitis**
117. The most common defect of femur in CDH is: → **A torsional defect of the upper femur**
118. The initial pathological change most commonly demonstrable in rheumatoid arthritis is → **Vasculitis**
119. The areas of most serious destruction in **early congenital syphilis is** → **Growth plates**
120. **Compression type arthrodesis** is most suitable for → **Ankle joint and knee joint**
121. Treatment of **clubfoot** is best begun on the → **Day of birth**
122. The **patella** is most often found at an abnormally high level in association with → **Recurrent dislocating patellae**
123. The most common site for **glomus tumour** is → **Phalanges**
124. Most commonly primary monoarticular rheumatoid arthritis is seen in → **Young females**

125. **Osteomas** most commonly originate in the → **Skull bone**
126. **Giant cell tumour** occurs most frequently around the → **Knee**
127. After **spinal cord injury,** the most important test indicating need for decompressive laminectomy is → **Queckenstedt test**
128. The most important sign to be noted in a patient of **head injury** is → **Changes in level of consciousness**
129. The **earliest laboratory finding in the fat embolism** is → **Lipuria**
130. The nerve most commonly involved in **causalgic reactions is the** → **Median nerve**
131. The nerve with the poorest prognosis for recovery after adequate surgical repair is the → **Sciatic nerve**
132. The most frequent associated injury with **fat embolization** is injury to the → **Hips**
133. A **bone graft** for the treatment of non-union is best obtained from → **Iliac crest of the patient**
134. Most commonly **"squared off patella"** is characteristic of → Haemophilia
135. Anterior spinal fusion in the thoracic area is most often performed because of → **Tuberculous infection**
136. **Serum alkaline phosphatase** is increased significantly in case of → **Rickets**
137. In **osteoarthritis (OA),** the earliest changes ensue in the → **Hyaline cartilage**
138. **Metastatic tumours to bone** are rarely found in the → Bone below knee or elbow
139. The **periosteal desmoid** is found most frequently on the → Posterior, distal femur
140. The most common complaint of a patient with **melorheostosis** is → **Transient pain**
141. **Osteomyelitis** is most commonlycaused by → *Staph. aureus*
142. **Congenital absence of a muscle** commonly most commonly affects → **Trapezius**

143. **Myositis ossificans** progressiva most commonly appear 1st in the posterior neck and → **Shoulder girdle**
144. The **most satisfactory biopsy method for bone lesion is** → Open biopsy guided by prior X-ray evaluation
145. A joint least likely to be affected by **chronic recurrent dislocation** is → **Knee joint**
146. The best treatment for **solitary bone cyst** is → Curettage beyond cavity walls and bone chips filling
147. **Multiple myeloma** tumour cells greatly resembles → **Plasma cells**
148. A most characteristic feature of **primary reticulum cell sarcoma of bone is** → Abundant cytoplasm and kidney-shaped nucleus
149. **Phantom bone disease** most commonly resembles histologically → Hamartoma
150. The early and most characteristic X-ray signs of **Sudeck's atrophy** are seen in the → Subchondral bone and site of old epiphyseal line
151. A **giant Baker's cyst** is most likely to be associated with → Thrombophlebitis
152. **Rupture of the intervertebral disc** most often occurs through the → Annulus fibrous away from midline
153. An **nonunion** following an **osteotomy** is most likely to be encountered in a patient with → Neurofibromatosis
154. The most important sign of **acetabular and hip dysplasia** in the **neonatal period** is → Limitation of abduction of the flexed thighs
155. The most commonly involved **cranial nerve in fracture** of the base of the skull is the → **7th cranial nerve**
156. **"Pelkan's spur"** is most commonly seen in → **Scurvy**

157. **Earliest radiological sign of rickets** is → Widening of epiphysis
158. **Recurrent dislocation** is most common in → Shoulder joint
159. The **scaphoid fracture** most prone to develop avascular necrosis is → Fracture through waist of scaphoid bone
160. Most common cause of **paraplegia of early onset tuberculosis of spine** is → Cold abscess pressing on the spinal cord
161. Most commonly **cortico-medullary differentiation** is absent in → Osteopetrosis
162. **Ring sequestrum** most commonly seen in → Lower part of bone after amputation
163. The best treatment for **fibrosarcoma of mid thigh** is → Hip disarticulation
164. Besides scaphoid, 2nd most common carpal bone to be fractured is → Lunate
165. Open reduction and internal fixation is almost always essential in → **Salter type IV fracture**
166. The treatment of choice in **psoriatic arthropathy is** → Methotrexate
167. The most acceptable angulation in fracture tibia is → **5 degree**
168. Most commonly **Froment's sign is positive due to paralysis of** → **Adductor pollicis**
169. Most commonly maximum weight can be applied/used in **skin traction is** → **Five to seven kg**
170. Most commonly **femoral head** in between **4 to 9 years** of age gets its blood supply from → **Only lateral epiphyseal vessels**
171. In **detecting bone infection** the best **scintiscan agent** is → **^{99m} Tc-MDP**
172. **Earliest bone metastasis** can be detected by → Radioisotope bone scan
173. **"Tumbling brick"** appearance in X-ray spine is seen most commonly in → **Neurosyphilis**

174. Most commonly in functional position of hand, metacarpo-phalangeal joints are held at flexion of	→	**Sixty degree**
175. **Cubitus valgus** deformity is mostly seen in	→	Fracture of lateral condyle of humerus
176. Most common C/P of **osteoporosis** is	→	Chronic backache
177. **Meralgia paraesthetica** is mostly due to compression of	→	Lateral cutaneous neve of thigh
178. **Ortolani's test** is most commonly done for cases of	→	CDH (congenital dislocation of hip)
179. **Acute osteomyelitis** in infants is best diagnosed by	→	History of high degree of suspicion
180. **Injury to extensor tendon of hand** is treated most commonly by	→	Primary suturing
181. **"Tom Smith arthritis"** most commonly involves	→	Femoral head
182. **Cubitus varus** is most commonly caused by	→	Supracondylar fracture
183. **Dupuytren's contracture** is more common in	→	**Alcoholics**
184. **Osteoblastic secondaries** are mostly seen in cases of	→	CA prostate
185. Treatment of coice for **Paget's disease** of bone is	→	Calcitonin
186. Earliest evidence of **healing in Rickets** is provided by	→	Radiological examination of growing end of bones
187. Most common cause of **septic arthritis** in young adults is	→	Gonococcal arthritis
188. **Osteochondritis dessicans** most commonly involves	→	**Knee joint**
189. Most common skeletal abnormality seen in **rickets** is	→	**Genu valgum**
190. **Medial semilunar cartilage** is most commonly damaged in knee joint because	→	Attached to tibial collateral ligament

191. **Ankylosing spondylitis,** most commonly are 1st seen in → **Sacro-iliac joint**
192. The most classical displacement in **Colles'fracture** is that the distal radial fragment is displaced → Upwards, backwards, and laterally
193. The most common condition associated with **Volkmann's ischaemic contracture** of **upper limb** is → Supracondylar fracture of the humerus
194. **Epiphysitis of the tibial tubercle** is most commonly given the nick name → Osgood-Schlatter disease
195. The most common causative organism in a **2 years old child** with **septic arthritis** is: → *Haemophilus influenzae*
196. The fracture most commonly associated with vascular injury in children is → **Fracture lower end of humerus**
197. Bone secondaries from **Breast CA** are most often → **Osteolytic**
198. **"Triple deformity of knee"** is most commonly seen in cases of → **Tuberculosis**
199. **Non-union of femoral shaft** is most commonly managed by → **Bone grafting and plating**
200. **Reflex sympathetic dystrophy** as a complication, is most commonly seen in → **Colles' fracture**
201. **In fracture neck femur** in a 64-year-old lady, the treatment of choice is → Prosthetic replacement arthroplasty of femoral head
202. Most common **Radial nerve injury** recovers with conservative management is → Neuropraxia
203. **Osteoclastoma** is most common in age group of → 20 to 40 years
204. Most commonly **Polio paralysis** differs from paralysis due to other causes in → **No sensory loss**
205. Most commonly **Syme's amputation** is contraindicated in → Diabetic foot
206. Most common **degenerative joint disease** is → Osteoarthritis

207. Most common cause of **recurrent shoulder dislocation** is	→	**Injury to humeral head**
208. The EMG change most characteristic of denervated muscle is	→	**Fibrillation potential**
209. Most common site of lesion in spinal muscular atrophy is	→	**Anterior horn cell**
210. The **surgery of choice in TB spine** is	→	**Hongkong procedure**
211. The most common source of bone and joint infection is from	→	**Haematogenous**
212. **Madelung's deformity** most commonly involves	→	**Wrist**
213. Most uncommon complication of osteomyelitis in adult human is	→	**Septic arthritis**
214. **DIC** following long bone fracture mostly ensues after	→	**Few days**
215. Most common cause of **reactive arthritis** is	→	**Shigella**
216. Most common cause of **kyphosis** in young adult males is	→	**Ankylosing spondylitis**
217. Most common fracture when a person falls from height is	→	**Fracture calcaneum**
218. Most commonly **pathological fracture** is seen in	→	**Secondaries in bone**
211. **Cubitus varus** deformity following supracondylar fracture is most commonly due to	→	**Medial angulation**
220. Most common cause of **pathological fracture** in a **6 years old child** is	→	**Solitary bone cyst**
221. **Chauffeurs fracture** most commonly involves	→	**Radius**
222. Treatment of choice in a young adult with **fracture neck femur** is	→	Close reduction and multiple screw fixation
223. Most common type of **supracondylar fracture** of **humerus** is	→	**Extension**
224. **Meniscal injuries** are most common with	→	**Rotation of knee**

225. **Anterior dislocation of shoulder** most commonly causes → **Axillary nerve palsy**
226. Most common deformity in **club foot** is → **Talipes equinovarus**
227. Joint most commonly involved in **monoarticular JRA (Juvenile Rheumatoid Arthritis) is** → **Knee joint**
228. Earliest EMG sign of reinnervation is appearance of → **Polyphasic, slow duration potential**
229. Most common tendon to rupture due to direct or indirect injury is → **Tendo-Achilles**
230. Most reliable clinical diagnostic feature of fracture is → **Crepitus**
231. Most common site of **solitary bony cyst is** → **Humerus upper end**
232. Most common type of **epiphyseal injury** is → **Type II**
233. Treatment of choice for **solitary bone cyst** is → **Curettage and bone grafting**
234. Bone haemangiomas are most often found in → **Vertebrae**
235. Most common site of **spine** affected by a **wedge compression fracture** is → **Thoraco-lumbar**
236. **Osteochondritis** presents at the earliest age (4 to 10 years) is: → Perthes's disease
237. The tumour most often causes **solitary metastasis** is → **Kidney**
238. Most common cause of **Pes cavus** is → Idiopathic
239. Most common site of **pigmented villonodular synovitis** is → **Knee**
240. The **type of fracture earliest to unite is** → **Spiral**
241. Nerve palsy most commonly seen in supracondylar fracture is → **Radial nerve**
242. **Double structural scoliotic curves** are most typically seen in → **Marfan's syndrome**
243. Most common cause of **genu varum** is → **Rickets**

244. Most common **primary malignant bone tumour** is → **Osteogenic sarcoma**
245. Most common site of skeletal TB is → **Spine**
246. Most common site of spinal TB is → **Thoracic**
247. Most common type of **spinal tuberculosis** is → **Paradiscal**
248. Most common site of disc prolapse is → **L4 and L5**
249. Most **common site of involvement of spine in** rheumatoid arthritis is → **Cervical**
250. Most common **carpal bone to fracture** is → **Scaphoid**
251. **Pseudoarthrosis** following triple arthrodesis is most common in → **Talonavicular joint**
252. Earliest **radiological sign of TB spine is** → **Decreased joint space**
253. Most **common cause of solitary vertebra plana** in **childhood** is → **Eosinophilic granuloma**
254. Most commonly **"spina ventosa"** results from → **TB**
255. Most commonly **Gaenslen's operation** is for → **Sacroiliac subluxation**
256. Carcinoma most likely to develop in **chronic osteomyelitis** is → **Squamous cell CA**
257. **Volkmann's ischemic contracture** most commonly associated with → **Supracondylar fracture of humerus**
258. The most important single sign in impending Volkmann's ischemic contracture is → **Stretch pain**
259. In **acute haematogenous osteomyelitis,** the earliest **radiological changes** in bone are seen in → **10 days**
260. Extensor tendon most often ruptured in **rheumatoid arthritis** is → **Extensor pollicis longus**
261. Most common site for **ivory osteoma** is → **Skull**
262. **"Melon seed bodies"** are most char-acteristic of → **Tubercular tenosinovitis**
263. Most important source of blood supply to the **femoral head** is → **Lateral epiphyseal artery**

264. Most common **late complication of acetabular fracture** is → **Avascular necrosis of femoral head**
265. Most common nerve palsy seen ina **fracture of midshaft of humerus** is → **Radial nerve**
266. In patient with **sickle cell anaemia** most **osteomyelitis** usually results from → **Salmonella typhi**
267. **Triple arthrodesis** is least likely to be successful in → **Calcaneous deformity**
268. **Earliest radiological sign** of **osteoarthritis** is → **Narrowing of joint space**
269. In **rheumatoid arthritis,** there is most primarily involvement of → **Synovial membrane**
270. Most commonly affected lower limb muscle in **Poliomyelitis** is → **Quadriceps femoris**
271. Joint least commonly involved in **Charcot's disease** is → **Wrist**
272. Hand joint most commonly involved in primary osteo-arthritis is → **Carpometa-carpal joint of thumb**
273. **Triple arthrodesis** for severe deformities of foot is done mostly at the age of → **10 years of age**
274. **Earliest radiological changes** of **Sudeck's atrophy** are charac-teristically seen in → **Subchondral bone and site of epiphyseal line**
275. **Fracture clavicle in a 10 years old child is best treated by** → **Figure of "8" bandage and an arm sling**
276. **Most accurate anthropometric index** useful in **Marfan's syndrome** is → **Upper segment lower segment ratio**
277. Finding of **phosphoethano-lamine in urine** is most pathognomic of → **Hypophospha-tasic rickets**
278. **Acute osteomyelitis** is most likely to spread to adjacent joint in → **Femur upper end**
279. **Pseudoarthrosis of tibia** is most often associated with → **Neurofibroma-tosis**
280. **Angular kyphosis** is most commonly produced by → **TB spine**

281. **Soft tissue sarcoma** most often invading the bone is → **Fibrosarcoma**
282. Bone most **commonly affected** by **Gaucher's disease** is → **Femur**
283. In **haemophilia,** the joints most commonly affected by **haemarthrosis** are → **Knee joint**
284. Most commonly a **benign neoplasm of bone** alone presents with pain is → **Osteoid osteoma**
285. The bone most **severely deformedin congenital talipes equinovarus** is → **Talus**
286. Most common site of a **glomus tumour affecting bone** is → **Phalanges**
287. Most commonly radiological appearance of **"brush skull"** is seen in → **Haemolytic anaemia**
288. In **Scruvy,** the "WIMBERGER LINE" is best seen in → **Patella**
289. Most common type of **"Spina bifida cystica"** is → **Myelocoele**
290. **Pure dislocations of vertebrae** are most commonly found in → **Cervical region**
291. Most common **bursa** involved in **Baker's cyst** is → **Semimembranosus**
292. **Earliest skeletal manifestation of rickets** is → **Craniotabes**
293. **Romanus lesion** is most characteristic of → **Ankylosing spondylitis**
294. Most common joint involved in **synovial osteochondromatosis** is → **Knee joint**
295. Ligament most commonly involved in **"sprained ankle"** is → Anterior talofibular ligament
296. Most common **fracture of childhood** is → **Clavicular fracture**
297. Most common complication of **fracture scaphoid** is → **Avascular necrosis**
298. Most commonly a carpal bone whose ossification center appears last is → **Pisiform**
299. **de Quervain's tenosynovitis** most commonly involves tendon ofand Abductor → Extensor pollicis brevis pollicis longus

300. **"Wandering acetabulum"** is seen most commonly in cases of → **Tuberculosis of hip**
301. **"Soap-bubble" appearance** on X-ray is seen most commonly in → **Osteoclastoma or germ cell tumour**
302. Most common site of **enchondroma** is → **Phalanges**
303. Most common **benign bone tumour** is → **Osteochondroma**
304. Treatment of choice in **impending Volkmann's ischemic contracture** is → **Slit the cast and perform a fasciotomy**
305. Most common cause of **calcification of articular cartilage of knee** is → **Pseudogout**
306. Most commonly **"Mallet finger"** results from → **Ruptured extensor mechanism at distal phalanx**
307. Most common **hormone that influences growth negatively** is → **GLUCOCORTICOIDS**
308. Most commonly **"Erlenmayer flask appearance" of femur is seen** in → **Gaucher's disease**
309. Most commonly **"laminated appearance" on X-ray is suggestive of** → **Ewing's sarcoma**
310. **Boxer's fracture** most commonly involves → **Fracture** 5th metacarpal head
311. Most common injury associated with fracture of pelvis is → **Injury to membranous urethra**
312. Most serious complication of a **compound fracture** is → **Infection**
313. **Bony ankylosis** is a most common sequelae to → Pyogenic arthritis
314. **"Gun-stock deformity"** most commonly results from malunited → Supracondylar fracture of humerus
315. Most common complication of **intertrochanteric fracture** is → **Malunion**
316. Most common mechanism of **ankle injury** is → **External rotation**

317. Large epiphyses with early epiphyseal closure is seen most commonly in → **Juvenile chronic arthritis (JCA)**
318. Most commonly **osteosclerosis** with ligamentous calcification is seen in → **Fluorosis**
319. Most commonly **"Trigger finger"** is usually associated with → **Rheumatoid tenosynovitis**
320. The results of **nerve repair** are poorest with → **Sciatic nerve**
321. Most commonly **anatomical position of 3 bony points** at **elbow** is not disturbed in → **Supracondylar fracture of humerus**
322. **Multiple "Punched out holes"** in skull are seen most commonly in → **Multiple myeloma**
323. Most commonly **ossification begins** in **foetus** during → **5th week of IUL**
324. Most commonly an enzyme found in osteoclast but not in osteoblast is → **Acid phosphatase**
325. Viscosity of synovial fluid mostly dependent on the concentration of → **Hyaluronic acid**
326. Eccentric subauricular radiolucent lesion in the end of long bone is mostly suggestive of → **Aneurysmal bone cyst**
327. Most commonly, the **"frog hand"** results from → **Deep palmar abscess**
328. **"Rocker bottom foot"** is mostly seen in → **Forcible correction of club foot**
329. Most commonly **recurrent talipes equinus** is due to failure of development of → **Peroneal muscles**
330. **Tri-radiate pelvis** is seen most commonly in → **Osteomalacia**
331. Mot commonly **"Allen test"** is done to assess → **Adequacy of radial or ulnar artery**
332. Most common site of **"stress fracture"** is → **2nd and 3rd metatarsal**
333. Treatment of choice in a child upto 3 years of age sustaining fracture **shaft femur** is → **Gallows traction**

334. Most commonly **"pointing index"** is seen in	→	**Median nerve lesion**
335. Best radiological view for diagnosing the fracture **Scaphoid bone is**	→	**Oblique view**
336. Most commonly **Brodie's abscess** is found in	→	**Long tubular bones**
337. Most commonly **symmetrical multiple spontaneous fractures occur** in	→	**Osteogenesis imperfecta**
338. Most common **complication of interscapular fracture neck of femur** is	→	**Nonunion**
339. **Osteomyelitis by haematogenous route** is most commonly caused by	→	***Staphylococcus aureus***
340. Most **common site of fracture clavicle is at the junction of**	→	**Medial 2/3rd and lateral 1/3rd**
341. **Best results of nerve suturing** are seen in	→	**Radial nerve**
342. **T.B. spine** mostly **initially begins** in	→	**Paradiscal body area**
343. **Keller's operation** most commonly involved excision of	→	**Proximal phalanx**
344. **Osteosarcoma** most commonly arises from	→	**Metaphysis**
345. Most common cause of **monoarthritis** is	→	**Septic arthritis**
346. **Osteoclastoma** most commonly occurs at	→	**Femur lower end**
347. Most common expansile osteolytic growth arising from the end of long bone after epiphyseal closure is	→	**Giant cell tumour**
348. **Myositis ossificans** is most commonly due to	→	Ossification of subperiosteal haematoma
349. Most commonly a fracture line visible on X-ray without sclerosis with no osteoporosis is clinically known as	→	**Slow healing**
350. **Osteosarcoma** most commonly arises from	→	**Lower end of femur**

351. Most commonly initial stage of clinical union of bone is equivalent to → **Woven bone**
352. Primary callus formation can be seen earliest on "X-ray" at → **15 to 30 days**
353. Most common cause of loose body in a joints → **Osteoarthritis**
354. **Osteoclastoma** (Giant cell tumour) arises most commonly from → **Epiphysis**
355. **Codman's triangle** due to lifting up of periosteum is found most commonly in → **Osteosarcoma**
356. **Dupuytren's contracture** of the hand most commonly starts in the → **Ring finger**

Chapter fourteen

Problem Oriented Orthopaedic Cases Seen in Clinical Practice

You Should Know

1. **Saloni** a 38 years old lady, gives a history of twisted strain and locking of the knee joint, the most likely diagnosis is→**Meniscal tear.**
2. **Shaukat Alam,** a 50 years old patient presented with a lusterless black lesion under the great toe nail. He has noticed the said lesion for three months. The most likely diagnosis is→**Malignant melanoma.**
3. A patient named **Raunaq** complains of severe low back pain with a sciatic distribution, aggravated by coughing, sneezing and straining, relieved by lying down is most characteristic of →**Ruptured intervertebral disc.**
4. **Rakesh,** a 25 years old male was having a chronic backache of 6 months duration. The pain was gradually increasing in severity and was worse at rest and in the morning on arising from bed. He had to slowly "work the pian out" and as these times the pain centered in his low back and radiated into his buttock and posterior left thigh. Physical examination revealed paraspinal muscle spasm with "flat back". All attempts at motion caused pain in the low back and into both legs. Genslen's sign is positive. The most likely diagnosis is **Rheumatoid spondylitis.**
5. **Al Quadir,** a 25-year-old male presented with a painful left foot. He gave a history of flat feet since the very childhood. The pain began at about the age 16 and became more gradually. At present any strenuous exercise would cause severe discom-

fort in the left foot. On physical examination, bilateral valgus feet was found but only the left foot was painful both during active or passive motion. Inversion of the foot was markedly limited and this caused the typical pain also. The most probable diagnosïs is →**Peroneal spastic flat foot.**

6. **Khensanilal,** a 30-year-old male fell from the roof of a house, landing on his feet in a couching position. He had immediate pain and inability to fully extend his left knee. In addition to patella, he might have sustained:
   - Tibial plateau
   - Femoral condyle
   - Os calcis
   - Posterior acetabulum
   - Vertebral body.
7. A person named **Kalimullah** falls from a height and the tensed up quadriceps acts on a partly flexed knee, it is likely to produce **fracture of the patella.**
8. **Sikander** a 60-year-old man stated that he had a painful left knee of 14 years duration with recent limitation of movement. On examination, the knee was found to be enlarged by firm tissue and a minimal amount of free fluid. Range of movement was 20° to 110° with creptius but very little pain. The tibia was enlarged in its upper one half and more prominence than the opposite tibia. X-ray showed sclerotic joint surfaces and joint space. Joint margins were remained by large osteophytic spurs. The left tibia was much denser with ill defined cortex and wider marrow space. The most probable diagnosis is→**Paget's disease.**
9. In a patient named **Komilla,** a severe open fracture complicated with sepsis would show the following metabolic changes during the 1st ten days following injury is:
   - Low 17-ketosteroid excretion
   - **Drop of corticosteroid in blood.**
10. **Anderson** a 25-year-old male had a hot, painful swelling just above the left knee, slowly enlarging

over the past from months. Weight loss and anaemia were also noted. Differential diagnosis includes:

- Osteomyelitis
- Osteogenic sarcoma.
- Malignant giant cell tumour.
- Ewing's sarcoma.

11. If a patient with Colle's fracture complains of numbness and paraesthesia of the thumb and index finger, it suggests→**Pressure on the median nerve.**
12. **Rinkoo**, a 14 years old girl has come to ortho OPD/emergency for the treatment of fracture in the upper limb. The attending doctor upon examination has found that there is a fracture of the olecranon and the fracture fragments are widely separated. The treatment of choice here is **reduction and internal fixation.**
13. **Karamchand** a 33 years old man sustained a midshaft humeral fracture after very slight exertion. X-ray showed the fracture to be through a bone cyst and other films showed widespread bone cysts in other bones. The abdominal film showed a kidney stone. The important diagnostic test is→**Urine calcium.**
14. In scurvy patient there is a zone of translucency on the metaphyseal side of the growth palate as seen by X-ray. This is known as **Zone of fracture-separation.**
15. A child named **Sudhanshu** was brought to emergency for pain following trauma to elbow region. The attending doctor has diagnosed this case a fracture of lateral condyle of humerus. In this situation, the most likely type of epiphyseal injury is →**Type IV**.
16. **Monu** a 10 years old child was brought to ortho-emergency for evaluation after fall from a height. The attending doctor has diagnosed it as a fracture clavicle. The clavicular fracture in a child is best treated by→**Figure of "8" bandage and an arm sling.**
17. **Paltu Mian** a 25 years old patient has brought to ortho OPD for fracture pelvis with associated ure-

thral injury. The first important step in management is treatment of **shock and haemorrhage.**

18. **Pintu**, a 27 years old patient was brought to ortho emergency following bullet injury in at upper extremity, there are signs of decreased perfusion and blood loss, one will do→**Immediate brachial artery exploration and repair.**
19. **Akbar Mian**, a 50 years old Muslim presents with bone pains and on investigation calcium and phosphorus levels in serum were found to be normal with elevation of serum alkaline phosphate. The probable diagnosis is→**Paget's disease.**
20. Fracture neck of femur with minimal displacement in 50 years old male is best treated by internal fixation.
21. Treatment of choice in a 5-year-old **Sonu** sustaining fracture shaft of femur at proximal one-third is sliding traction in **Thomas's splint.**
22. **Gazala,** a child with upper brachial plexus injury avoids abduction and adduction of digits. The muscles involved are **Interossei.**
23. **Sukant** an infant has fever and severe pain in hip joint. On aspiration, pus is obtained and Gram stain shows that there is ***Staphylococcus***. Best form of treatment to be given here is **operative drainage.**
24. **Ghasitta,** an elderly labourer while lifting heavy weight developed sudden quadriplegia. One should look for **atlantoaxial dislocation.**
25. **Mannmeet Singh** a middle aged male fell from a height presents with shortening of lower limb, internal rotation and tenderness and a mass in gluteal region. The most likely diagnosis is→**"Posterior dislocation of hip".**
26. In a patient named **Tunna mian,** in fixed adduction deformity of hip, anterior superior iliac spine is at higher level than normal. It can be made level with the opposite anterior superior iliac spine by →**adduction of the affected limb.**
27. In a 6 years old child **Rinkoo,** X-ray of long bones shows metaphyseal radio-opaque line, generalized decalcification (ground glass appearance) with linear translucencies is→**Scurvy.**

28. A child named **Kalloo**, 10 years old is brought to ortho OPD for one-year-old posterior dislocation of hip. Treatment of choice in this situation is→**Leave it alone.**
29. After 10 weeks of posterior dislocation of hip in a 20 years old **Rajan Pillay.** The treatment is skeletal traction to release muscle contracture and surgery and **correct the dislocation.**
30. **Rajoo Singh** a 33 years old male patient develops compartment syndrome (swelling, pain and numbness) following manipulation and plaster for fracture of both bones of leg. The best treatment in to do **operative decompression of fascial compartment.**
31. Subsequent to a fall, a 20 years old **Shaukat** is unable to lift his injured upper limb. On inspection, the normal rounded contour of the shoulder is found to have been lost; the upper arm appears longer on the injured side of the acromion is prominent. The most likely diagnosis is→**Anterior dislocation of the shoulder.**
32. **Renuka** a 36 years old mother of four children has been noticing a hard painless swelling in front of the neck during the past 8 months, gradually increasing in size. On coming down the stairs, she suddenly felt excruciating pain in the left hip and fell down and could not get up any more. The most likely diagnosis is pathological fracture of upper end of femur.
33. In a patient named **Sulekha,** ape thumb deformity, pointing index finger, inability to oppose the thumb and flex the terminal phalanx of thumb, index and middle fingers suggest paralysis of→**Median nerve.**
34. **Kaliva**, a known patient with renal stone disease developed pathological fractures along with abdominal pain and certain psychiatric symptoms. He should be investigated for →**Hyperparathyroidism.**
35. **Hausain** an 8 years old boy presents with progressive swelling around the knee joint of two months duration following mild trauma. Local ex-

amination reveals an irregular bony swelling over the upper end of tibia, with raised local temperature and of variable consistency and ill-defined margins. The most likely diagnosis is→**Osteogenic sarcoma.**

36. **Rahman Mian,** a man who cuts himself across the palm of the right hand over the distal palmar areas three hours before presenting himself at the casualty. On examinations, he is unable to flex the middle and distal joints of the ring finger. Extension is normal. There is no sensory loss. Besides antibiotics and antitetanus globulin, the most appropriate treatment for this patient would be→**Primary suture of flexor digitorum sublimis and flexor digitorum profundus tendons.**

37. **Ramaiyaa** a 60 years old lady presents at the OPD clinic with an old malunited Colles' fracture of the left wrist with complaining of disfiguration of the wrist but no functional disability. The most appropriate course of management would be **reassurance and leave it alone.**

38. **Tung-Sung**, a 12-year-old boy fell down and suffered acute pain in the shoulder. Examination revealed tenderness and swelling over the upper third of humerus. X-ray revealed a pathological fracture through a translucent area in the metaphysis with the bone expanded in fusiform manner with thin cortex and no periosteal reaction. The translucent area extended upto the epiphyseal plate. The most likely diagnosis is→**Solitary bone cyst.**

39. **Tom Louis**, a person reports to ortho OPD with vertebral fracture, hemiplegia and urinary retention, in such situation the emergency measure to be taken in urethral catheterization.

40. **Fulkli** a 9 years old child has suffering from joint pain is brought to ortho OPD for further evaluation and treatment. The attending doctor after thorough examination and investigation diagnosed her a case of rheumatoid arthritis with proteinuria and oedema. The above clinicopathologic findings is suggestive of **Rheumatoid nephropathy.**

41. **Moin Mian** a 29 years old male has been complaining of pain in right side to buttock, posterior thigh, calf and lateral aspect of foot for 6 months. Cough and straining tended to aggravate the pain. There is no sensory defect and no urinary complaints. The most probable diagnosis is→**Herniation of lumbar intervertebral disc.**
42. **Harry Gold** a 16 years old boy has gradually developed muscle weakness accompanied by muscular pain on movement. There is associated erythematous skin eruption and diplopia. This suggests→**Dermatomyositis.**
43. In a patient with known T.B. of the spine the most constant sign of imminent paraplegia due to pressure on the cord is→**Clonus.**
44. **Kehu-Mian**, a 35 years old man enters your office complaining of hip pain. X-ray film shows that he has aseptic necrosis of femoral head. The most likely time when the patient would become symptomatic with this condition could be **when crescent sign is present on X-ray films.**
45. **Cheddilal** a 30 years old man comes to your clinic complaining that on running in a lateral direction or cutting, he has a strange feeling that he loses control of his knee, otherwise his knee feel normal. Your initial impression would be rotatory instability. The best way to test from impression would be **check anterior drawer sign in 90° flexion and 150° of external rotation.**
46. **Pradeep Yadav** a 45 years old man is found to have a L4 to L5 disc rupture and surgery is performed to correct this lesion. The patient does well for 6 months until pain returns in the back and he begins having headache and stiff neck. On physical examinations, the following would be a significant diagnostic finding→**is questionable fluctuant mass in the area of prior surgery.**
47. **Sunita**, a 50 years old female was seen complaining of a severe aching pain in upper dorsal spine of one week's duration. Neurologically she was normal except for pain radiating around her chest in the mid-area. Temperature was 38°C. X-rays

revealed a narrowing and wedging of T4, T5 disc space and partial collapse of T4 with erosion of the superior end plate of T5. The most likely diagnosis is→**Pyogenic infection.**

48. **Mallu Khan** a 60 years old man complained of moderate pain of a gradually enlarging swelling in his right knee of four months duration. There was no history of trauma. It had become worse over the past month. Examination revealed the knee to be swollen with only moderate reaction in the knee joint as a mildly thickened synovia but no palpable free joint fluid. The main finding was a distension of the prepatellar bursa by a doughy mass. Range of knee motion was 0° to 110° and painful only in full flexion. The overlying skin was roughened but otherwise of normal colour and was not warmer than the other knee. The most probable diagnosis is→**Tuberculosis.**

49. **Urmilla Singh** a 21 years old female presents with a history general malaise and bouts of marked irritability. She has been seen on several previous occasions with the same complaints but without any pathological findings. On this occasion, X-rays revealed a diffuse, scattered snowflake quality of increased densities in both kidneys. A positive urinary sulkowitch was present. X-rays of long bones showed only a generalised lack of cortical sharpness especially at the diaphyseal, metaphyseal junctions. The patient while undergoing evaluation, suddenly went into shock and the blood pressure falls. At this time, a blood calcium/phosphorus report is returned to reading serum calcium 15 mg% and phosphorus, 28 mg%. The probable diagnosis is **hyperparathyroid crisis.**

50. **Laddu Mian,** a 64 years old male presents complaining of chronic aching pain in both hips and knees. Examination reveals a patient with a disproportionate anatomy. His head appears larger than normal in proportion to his total stature. His spine shows a kyphotic deformity and his legs are bowed both laterally and anteriorly. He insists on further questioning that he had none of these de-

formities at age thirty and there is no history of trauma. The most probable diagnosis is→**Paget's disease.**

51. An one-year-old child **Dibya** with a bowed leg of an anterior-tibial variety also showed a cystic change in mid-tibial area. The most likely diagnosis to be considered would be→**Neurofibromatosis**
52. **Fang Sui,** a 38 years old man limped into emergency room and stated he believed he had been kicked in the posterior aspect of his leg during a game of hand-ball. He had an immediate sharp pain and tenderness at the junction of middle and distal heel of leg. He had weak plantar flexion of his foot accompanied by pain in the calf. The most probable diagnosis is→**Rupture of Achilles tendon.**
53. **Debu** an 18 months old male child was presented by his mother because he was slower in beginning to walk than his siblings. He would crawl and put solid foods into his mouth at meals, but did not talk. Physical examination revealed an obvious normally developed child who was alert and would crawl with a swimming motion. All joints were normal and had a full range of motion. Sensations were apparently intact. Reflexes were normal in upper limbs and slightly more hyperactive than usual in the lower limbs. Further questioning revealed the child had been hospitalized for respiratory difficulties 5 days beyond the mother's discharge at the time of birth. The most probable diagnosis is→**Cerebral palsy (CP).**
54. **Sukriti** a 23 years old girl was seen after 4 days of illness. She had an onset of headache, malaise and vomiting. The headache became her chief complaint after 24 hours with an associated stiff neck. She developed weakness about the shoulder 70 years after onset and when first examined was drowsy and cooperated half heartedly. Physical examination showed weakness in the left deltoid and scapular muscles and weakness of the right triceps and hand grip. Temperature was 38.5°C.

Reflexes were absent in the upper extremity but present in lower extremity. Sensation was normal to gross testing. The most likely diagnosis is→**Poliomyelitis.**

55. In a patient named **Maqbool**, two hours after application of the plaster cast for supracondylar fracture, the patient comes back to emergency room with a complaint of severe pain in the hand. Examination revealed swelling of the fingers and cyanosis. The best course would be to **cut open the entire plaster cast immediately**.
56. **Sudhanshu** a 15 years old boy presents with a chief complain of pain in the knees. About 6 months prior to this examination the patient had injured his left knee while playing football. Immediately after this injury the boy experienced severe pain in left knee and a moderate degree of soft tissue swelling of this joint. The injury responded to conservative treatment and the patient returned to athletics 3 weeks later. The boy remained in good health until 2 months before, at which time he experienced pain in both knees while climbing stairs. The pain appeared to be increasing in severity as time progressed. At the time of this examination pain was elicited in both knees on kneeling and on active extension of the knees against resistance. Soft tissue swelling and pain were localized to the region of the tibial tubercles. X-rays revealed tibial tubercle soft tissues anterior to the tubercles. The most likely diagnosis is→**Osgood-Schlatter's disease.**
57. **Shrawan Pandey**, a 21 years old man presents with a 6 months history of acting and stiffness in the sacroiliac joints. At first the patient regarded this as a result of "two soft a mattress" because the backache occurred in the morning and seemed to disappear with activity. During the past month he noted sciatic radiation of the pain and backache when sitting for periods in one position. The patient claimed that the pain appeared to be extending upward along the vertebral column. On

examination, this patient has severe paraspinal muscle spasm. In addition there was a loss of the normal cervical and lumbar lordosis; indeed the entire back appeared kyphotic. The most likely diagnosis is→**Marie-Strumpell spondylitis.**

58. **Botu Mian** a 12 years old boy is admitted to the hospital with a chief complain of "severe pain in the left leg". History reveals that one week prior to admission the patient had been treated for scarlet fever. He now presents with the following clinical features. (i) restlessness and headache (ii) vomiting (iii) general appearance of severe illness (iv) rapid pulse rate (v) temperature of 104°C (vi) severe pain in the left leg. The WBC count is 21,000 per cmm. The left knee joint is extremely tender to touch and manipulation. Point tenderness is localized to the distal end of the femur. The neighboring joint can be manipulated without increasing the pain. No swelling is found in any other joints. X-rays including film of the left knee joint reveal no abnormalities. The most likely diagnosis is→**Acute osteomyelitis.**

59. **Mano Mian**, a 60 years old man presents with a chief complain of pain in the left knee for 8 months. On examination, there is no elevation of temperature and no constitutional symptoms. The patient remarked that "the knee is stiff but seemed to get better when moving around. However, the joint became swollen and pain appeared to be increasing in severity. The examiner finds on moving the knee joint a sensation of crunching and harsh grating sensation. The only other positive finding on physical examination is some evidence of generalized arteriosclerosis. X-ray examination of the left knee joint are reported on showing areas of degeneration and osteophyte formation. The most likely diagnosis is→**osteoarthritis.**

60. **Aslam** a 15 years old boy presented with painful swelling over the left shoulder. Radiography of the shoulder showed an osteolytic area with stippled calcification over the proximal humeral epiphysis.

Biopsy of the lesion revealed a immature fibrous matrix with scattered giant cells. The most likely diagnosis is→**Chondroblastoma**.

61. **Rustam Ali**, a 46 years old, known alcoholic, presented with pain in the dorsal spine. On examination, there is tenderness at the dorso-lumbar junction. Radiography shows destruction of the 12th dorsal vertebra with loss of disc space between D12-L1 vertebrae. The most probable diagnosis is→**Pott's spine.**
62. **Nellu Mian**, a 59 years old man sustained posterior dislocation of left hip in an accident. Dislocation was reduced after 3 days. He started complaining pain in left hip after 6 months. X-ray of the investigation at this stage will be→**MRI of hip.**
63. **Nirmal,** a 30 years old man involved in a fisticuffs, injured his middle finger and noticed slight flexion of DIP joint. X-rays were normal. The most appropriate management at this stage is **splint the finger in hyperextension.**

Note: This is a case of Mallet finger.

64. **Kalgi**, a 1½-year-old child holding her father's hand slipped and fell but did not let go of her father's hand. After then, she continued to cry and hold the forearm in pronated position and refused to move the affected extremity. The management at this stage includes: **Supinate the forearm.**

*Note: This is a case of **Pulled elbow.***

65. A young lady named **Kamla** met with an accident and had mild quadriparesis. Her lateral X-ray cervical spine revealed C_5-C_6 fracture dislocation. The best line of management is **cervical traction followed by instrument fixation.**

Note: Traction is best applied through Cone's or Barton's calipers.

66. **Mast Maula** a 45 years old was given steroids after renal transplant. After 2 years he had difficulty in walking and pain in both hips. The most

likely cause here is →**Avascular necrosis of femur head.**

> ***Note:*** *It is best diagnosed by MRI scan.*

67. **T.P. Sharma** a 30-year-old man had road-traffic accident and sustained femoral fracture. Two days later he developed sudden breathlessness. The most probable cause may be→**Fat embolism.**

> ***Note:*** *In fact, fracture femur depicts as a classic case of fat embolism. The prognosis is very poor.*

68. **Sakina** an elderly female > 50 years presents with walking/standing not possible. There is pain, spasmodic adduction with slight external rotation. There is shortening in limb length. Radiology is confirmatory. The most likely **complications** seen here is non union, malunion, shortening, stiff hip, avascular necrosis and degenerative arthrosis, etc.

Chapter fifteen

Last Moment Revision in Orthopaedics

You Should Know

1. **Direct impact on bone** will produce a **transverse** fracture.
2. **"Whip-lash" injury** is caused due to **acute hyperextension of the spine.**
3. **On 3 phase ^{99m}Tc-MDP** bone scan, the lesions showing least osteoblastic activity is **fibrous cortical defect.**
4. A 12 years old girl Neena complains of pain persisting in her leg for several weeks with a low grade fever. A radiograph reveals a mass in the diaphyseal region of the left femur with overlying cortical erosion and soft tissue extension. A biopsy of the lesion shows numerous small round cells, rich in PAS positive diastase sensitive granules. The most likely and consisting histological diagnosis is **Ewing's sarcoma.**

*Note: **Onion peel appearance** of Ewing's sarcoma is better demonstrated by CT/MRI scan than ordinary X-ray films.*

5. **Regarding metaphysis:**
   - It is the most vascular part of bone.
   - Growth activity is maximally seen here (active growth zone).
   - It is the commonest site of osteomyelitis in children only.
   - It is the region favouring haematogenous spread of infection.

> ***Note: Diaphysis** is the strongest part of bone not the metaphysis.*

6. **Injury to radial nerve** in lower part of spiral groove leaves extension at elbow joint intact.
7. The injury to **radial nerve** ensues most commonly in the distal part of the spiral groove, beyond the origin of the nerves to the triceps and the anconeus.
8. All muscles supplied by **radial nerve** except triceps and anconeus are paralysed in high radial nerve palsy.
9. **Avascular necrosis** is seen in fracture femoral neck, talus and scaphoid bone but not in **calcaneus bone.**
10. Sciatic nerve palsy may occur in **posterior hip dislocation.**
11. Common problems seen in **posterior hip dislocation** include:
    - Injury to sciatic nerve:
    - Avascular necrosis of femoral head
    - Myositis ossificans (MO)
    - Osteoarthritis (OA)
12. A 30 years old male was brought to the casualty following a road traffic accident. His physical examination revealed that his right lower limb was short, internally rotated, and flexed and abducted at the hip. The most likely diagnosis is **posterior dislocation of hip.**

> ***Note:** In **posterior dislocation of hip,** the classic deformity of flexion, adduction and internal rotation along with shortening is seen.*

13. **Osteomalacia** is associated with increase in **osteoid maturation time.**
14. A classical expansive **lytic bone lesion** in the transverse process of vertebra is seen in **aneurysmal bone cyst.**
15. **"Kienbock's disease"** is due to avascular necrosis of **lunate bone.**

16. **Walking downhill** will be difficult to perform for a patient with an anterior cruciate deficient **knee joint.**
17. In **anterior cruciate ligament injury,** there may be difficulty in descending stairs or squatting.
18. In **isolated posterior cruciate ligament injury,** instability is felt only in climbing stairs.
19. **Crush syndrome** includes—Crushing of muscles, myohemoglobinuria and acute tubular necrosis.

> *Note: It is not associated with **bleeding diathesis.***

20. A 40 years old man was repairing his wooden shed. By afternoon he felt that the hammer has becoming heavier and heavier. He felt pain in lateral side of elbow and also found that squeezing water out of sponge hurt his elbow. The most likely diagnosis from the history is **Tennis elbow.**

> *Note: It is a painful condition of lateral epicondyle involving the muscles **extensor carpiradialis longus and brevis.***

21. **Activities that causes tennis elbow include:**
    - Squeezing clothes.
    - Carrying suitcase
    - Using screw driver
    - Backhand smash with flexed elbow in Tennis player.
22. An 11-year-old boy presented with the complains of pian in the right arm near the shoulder. X-ray examination revealed an expansile lytic lesion in the upper one-third of humerus. The most likely diagnosis is **unicameral bone cyst.**
23. **The classical flexion and rotation deformities at hip and knee joints** as a sequelae of poliomyelitis are due to the contraction of **Tensor fascia lata.**
24. The **ilio-tibial tract contracture** causes:
    - Lumbar lordosis.
    - Pelvic obliquity.
    - External tibial torsion.
    - Flexion of hip and abduction of leg.
    - Genuvalgum and flexion of knee.

> ***Note:*** *These above actions of iliotibial tract is solely due to contracture of the muscle* ***tensor fascia lata.***

25. **"O" Donoghue triad** consists of injury to medial collateral ligament, medial meniscus and anterior cruciate ligament.
26. The most reliable test for an acutely injured knee of a 27 years old athlete is **"Lachmann test".**

> ***Note:*** *Lechmann test is more reliable than anterior Drawer test.*

27. In **athletes,** most **common ligamentous injury** at **knee** is anterior cruciate ligament followed by **meniscus.**
28. **Medial meniscus of knee joint** is injured more often than the lateral meniscus because the medial meniscus is relatively **less mobile.**
29. **Regarding meniscal injury**
    - "Bucket handle tears" are the most common injury.
    - Being avascular once menisci torn does not heal at all.
    - Presents as recurrent attacks of pain and locking of knee joint.
    - No swelling at the time of injury but later on reactive sympathetic effusion ensues, so become swollen.
    - History of sudden locking and unlocking with a click is diagnostic.
    - To detect tear **Mc Murray** and **Apley test** are done.
30. The operative procedure known as **"micro-fracture"** is done for **osteochondral defect of femur.**
31. A 30-year-old male with **nephrotic syndrome** complains of pain in right hip joint of 2 months duration. Thc movcmcnts at thc hip arc frcc but painful terminally. The most likely diagnosis is **avascular necrosis of femoral head.**

32. The most commonly affected component of the **lateral collateral ligament** complex in an "**ankle sprain**" is the anterior components.
33. The **stability of the ankle joint** is maintained by deltoid ligament, lateral ligament and shape of the superior talor articular surface.

> ***Note: Spring ligament** is not helpful in ankle joint stability.*

34. A pole vaulter had a fell during pole vaulting and had paralysis of the arm. In this set up, the investigation gives the best recovery prognosis is **Electromyography.**
35. In a patient with a history of burning pian localized to the plantar aspect of the foot, the D/d must include **tarsal tunnel syndrome.**
36. An elderly woman was admitted with a fracture of the neck of right femur which failed to unite. On examination, an avascular necrosis of the head of femur was noted. The condition would have resulted most probably from the damage to retinacular branches of **circumflex femoral arteries.**
37. **Ideal treatment of a fracture** which is not uniting is **compression plates** and **bone grafting.**
38. **Comminuted fracture of head of radius** in a child is treated by excision of head.
39. **Trendelenburg's test** mainly tests the action of gluteus medius.
40. **Avascular necrosis** following fracture is commonly seen in **Talus.**
41. Inversion/eversion takes place mainly at **subtalor joint.**
42. Most common complication of extracapsular fracture of neck of femur is **malunion.**
43. Most common type of **dislocation of hip** seen in **posterior.**
44. **Complete claw hand** results from injury due to **median + ulnar nerve injury.**
45. A 44 years old man presented with acute onset of low backache radiating to the right lower limb. Examination revealed SLR $< 40^\circ$ on the right side,

weakness of extensor hallucis longus on the right side, sensory loss in the 1st web space of the right foot and brisk knee jerk. The most likely diagnosis is **prolapsed intervertebral disc.**

46. A woman of 45, a known cause of **Pemphigus vulgaris** on a regular treatment with controlled primary disease presented with **pain** in the **right hip** and **knee.** Examination revealed no limb length discrepancy but the patient has tenderness in the **Scarpa's triangle** and limitation of adduction and internal rotation of the right hip joint as compared to the other side. The most probable diagnosis is →**Avascular necrosis of femoral head.**
47. A 27 years old male known epileptic, presented following a seizure with pain in the right shoulder region. Examination revealed that the right upper limb was adducted and internally rotated and the movements could not be performed. The most likely diagnosis is **posterior dislocation of shoulder.**
48. A 10 years old boy presenting with a cubitus varus deformity and a history of trauma 3 months back on clinical examination has the **preserved 3 bony points relationship of the elbow.** The most probable diagnosis is **malunited supracondylar fracture of humerus.**

> *Note: Three bony points relationship at elbow is disturbed in intercondylar fracture, fracture medial epicondyle and fracture lateral epicondyle.*

49. **C_A prostate** usually produce **osteoblastic secondaries.**
50. **Renal cell C_A** produces **osteolytic lesion.**
51. A 33 years old man presented with a slowly progressive swelling in the middle one-third of his right tibia. X-ray examination revealed multiple sharply demarcated **radiolucent lesions separated by areas of dense** and **sclerotic bone.** Microscopic examination of a biopsy specimen revealed islands of epithelial cell in a fibrous stroma. The most probable diagnosis is **ADAMANTINOMA.**

52. An army recruit, smoker and 6 months into training started complaining of pain at posteromedial aspect of both legs. There was acute point tenderness and the pain was aggravated on physical activity. The most likely diagnosis in **Stress fracture**.
53. In some old fractures, cartilaginous tissue forms over the fractured bone ends with a cavity in between containing clear fluid. This condition is called as **pseudoarthrosis.**
54. **Aseptic loosening in cemented total hip replacement** occurs as a result of hypersensitivity response to high density polyethylene debris.
55. In **fracture of olecranon,** excision of proximal fragment is indicated in:
    - Old ununited fractures
    - Non-articular fracture.
    - Elderly patients.
    - Open fractures.

> *Note: It is not done in fracture extending to coronoid process.*

56. **Tuberculous spine** commonly affects the vertebral body, lamina and pedicle but rarely spinous process.
57. Following can be the complications of a **malunited Colles fracture:**
    - Reflex sympathetic dystrophy.
    - Carpal tunnel syndrome.
    - Carpal instability.

> *Note: It is not seen as rupture of flexor pollicis longus tendon but in extensor pollicis longus.*

58. The **management of fat embolism** includes O_2 therapy heparinisation, low mol. wt. dextran.

> *Note: It does not require pulmonary embolectomy.*

59. **Management plan for osteogenic sarcoma** of the lower end of femur must include: Chemotherapy and limb salvage surgery + chemotherapy.
60. **Regarding chondroblastoma:**
    - Male to female ratio is 2:1.

- Age mostly affects teen age groups.
- Has a strict predilection for epiphysis and apophysis.
- It produces a characteristic chicken wire pattern of mineralization.
- Non-neoplastic osteoclastic giant cells are found.
- Radiologically spotty calcification is seen.

61. **Regarding giant cell tumour:**
    - Seen in 20 to 40 years age group.
    - Characteristically exhibits "soap bubble appearance" on X-ray.
    - There is no calcification within the tumour.
62. **Regarding chondromyxoid fibroma:**
    - Starts in metaphyseal region.
    - Affects 20 to 30 years age group.
    - Osteoclastic type giant cell presents.
    - X-rays demonstrate an eccentric geographic lucency that is very well delineated from the adjacent bone by a rim of sclerosis.
63. The most common **extrarenal involvement** in autosomal dominant (AD) polycystic kidney disease (PKD) is **Hepatic cysts.**
64. **Hypercalcemia** may be seen in:
    - Prolonged immobilization.
    - Sarcoidosis.
    - Multiple myeloma.

> *Note: It is not seen in **tumour lysis syndrome** rather may cause **Hypocalcemia.***

65. **Deep venous thrombosis (DVT) and pulmonary embolism** are the most common thrombotic condition seen in patients with cancer.
66. The most **common cancer associated with the thromboembolic episodes** include **lung, pancreas, GIT, breast, ovary, genitourinary cancers, lymphomas** and **brain tumours.**
67. The **diagnosis of DVT** in patients with cancer is made by IMPEDENCE PLETHYSMOGRAPHY or **bilateral compression USG** of the leg veins.

> ***Note:*** *Elevation of* ***D-dimer*** *is not as predictive of DVT in patients with cancer as it is in patients without cancer.*

68. Patients with cancer and a diagnosis of **DVT** or **pulmonary embolism** should be treated initially with IV **fractionated heparin** or low mol. wt. **heparin** for at least **5 days** and warfarin started within **1 or 2 days.**

> ***Note:*** *Patients with proximal DVT and a relative contraindication to heparin anticoagulation (haemorrhagic brain metastasis or pericardial effusion) should be considered for placement of a filter in the IVC (Greenfield filter) to prevent pulmonary embolism.*

69. Patients with **cancer** who undergo a major surgical procedure should be considered for **heparin prophylaxis** or **pneumatic boots** to prevent thromboembolism.
70. **Breast cancer** patients undergoing chemotherapy and patients with implanted catheters should be considered for prophylaxis (1 mg warfarin per day) to prevent thromboembolism, etc.
71. The **bone** receives 10% of the **cardiac output.**
72. Remodelling of bone is accomplished by two distinct cell types: **Osteoblasts** produce bone matrix and osteoclasts resorb the matrix.
73. **Measurement of bony mass** involves dual energy X-ray absorptiometry (DXA), Single energy X-ray absorptiometry (SXA), quantitative CT and ultrasound (USG).

> ***Note:*** *Of which* ***DXA*** *is* ***highly accurate*** *and of choice at most of the centres around the world.*

74. Drugs causing generalised osteoporosis (ring) in adults.
    - Glucocorticoid
    - Cyclosporine
    - Cytotoxic drugs
    - Anticonvulsant

- Excessive alcohol
- Lithium
- Aluminium
- Gn RH agonists
- Heparin

75. **CAT scan** is primarily used to measure the **spine**, and peripheral **CT** is used to measure bone in the **forearm** and **tibia**.

> *Note: Research into the use of CT for measurement of **hip** pathology is going on.*

76. A **susceptibility locus for Paget's disease** has been mapped to **chromosome 18q 21-22**—a region that contains the gene for a rare Paget disease called as **familial expansile osteolysis.**
77. **Pamidronate** is the only biphosphonate currently approved for IV use in **Paget's disease**.
78. The **incidence of osteosarcomas** in **Paget's disease** is day by day decreasing owing to more effective management of the case.
79. **Osteoclast-rich benign giant cell tumours** may develop in areas adjacent to **pagetic bone** and respond to **glucocorticoid treatment.**
80. Suspected areas of malignant transformation are best distinguished from pagetic bone by **CT** or **MRI.**

> ***Note:** Definitive diagnosis of malignancy requires **bone biopsy.***

81. Tumour typically affects the epiphysis of a long bone includes:
    - Osteoclastoma (Giant cell tumour)
    - Chondroblastoma.
82. Tumour arises from the metaphysis includes:
    - Osteosarcomas.
    - Bone cyst (Unicameral/Aneurysmal).
    - Chondroma/Osteochondroma.
    - Endrondroma.
    - Chondromyxoid fibroma.
    - Primary chondrosarcoma.
    - Fibrous cortical defect.

83. Tumours originating from diaphysis:
    - Ewing's tumour.
    - Admantinoma.
    - Multiple myeloma.
    - Osteoid osteoma.
84. Dequervain's disease classically affects the extensor pollicis brevis and abductor pollicis longus muscles.

> ***Note:*** *In Dequervain's tenosynovitis Finkelstein test is +ve.*

85. The pathognomonic F/O Rheumatoid arthritis is→Rheumatoid nodules.
86. Heberden's nods are found in DIP joints in osteoarthritis (OA).
87. Bony enlargement of DIP joints are seen in case of OA has been given the name→**Bouchard's nodes.**
88. In trigger finger the level of tendon sheeth constriction is found at the level of→Metacarpo-phalangeal joint.

> ***Note:*** *It most commonly affects 3rd/4th finger.*

89. The most common sequelae of tuberculous spondylitis in an adolescent in Bony ankylosis.

> ***Note:*** *Fibrous ankylosis is seen in healed T.B. joints except spine where bony ankylosis ensues.*

90. The most useful radio pharmaceutical for skeletal imaging in ^{99m}Tc MDP.
91. Regarding fracture of Atlas vertebra:
    - Jefferson fracture is the most common type.
    - Atlanto occipital fusion may sometimes be needed.
    - CAT scans should be done for diagnosis.
    - MRI scan is more useful.
92. Subtrochanteric fractures of femur may be treated by following methods:
    - Ender's nail.
    - Skeletal traction on Thomas' splint.

> ***Note: Smith Paterson nail*** *is used for fracture femoral neck while supracondylar fracture need* ***condylar blade plate****.*

93. The gold standard for the diagnosis of osteoporosis is DEXA.
94. The choice investigation for evaluation of suspected Perthes' disease is **MRI scan.**
95. The common sits involved by pelvic fracture includes:
    - Pubic rami.
    - Alae of ileum.
    - Acetabula.

> ***Note:*** *Ischial tuberositis fracture are very much rare indeed.*